Letters of Hope and Wisdom for Brain Injury Survivors

Letters of Hope and Wisdom for Brain Injury Survivors: Thoughts from a Counselor offers a personal, informal, and spiritual perspective on how to manage the multiple issues related to brain injury. Written by a counselor who draws on firsthand experiential testimonies and insights, each chapter offers a personal letter to the survivor addressing the various issues stemming from a brain injury, along with practical applications suggested for recovery.

The book offers a general overview of brain injury and how each part of the brain may be affected. Mental health issues such as depression, anxiety, anger, fear, post-traumatic stress, and grief are described from the perspectives of both the survivor and the family members, and the book also includes strategies on improving self-esteem and gaining new purpose after a brain injury. Additionally, practical coping skills are explained such as how to deal with sensory overload, adjusting the pace of life, and managing family events. Each chapter also offers a homework section that gives the reader additional exercises to complete.

It is valuable reading for brain-injured survivors seeking holistic wellbeing, and their family members to help them navigate what lies before them. It also serves as an additional source of therapy for clinicians, counselors, and upper-level graduate students.

Deana Adams is President of Hope After Brain Injury, a nonprofit organization dedicated to encouraging, educating, and equipping those on the brain injury journey. She hosts annual conferences and facilitates monthly support groups. As Executive Director of Hope Behavioral Health, Dr. Adams also offers counseling to survivors and families with brain injury.

'Letters of Hope and Wisdom is a treasure trove of practical advice, emotional support, and spiritual guidance...This book will be a trusted and valuable companion for those affected by brain injury.'
   –**Michael S. Arthur**, author of *Embracing Hope After Traumatic Brain Injury: Finding Eden* (Routledge 2022)

'When our family faced a crisis with a concussion, Dr. Deana Adams was a careful guide and a wise encouragement for the challenges we faced. Her writing and counsel gave hope and insight into the mysteries of healing.'
   –**Lorna Dueck**, Media Consultant, LornaDueckCreative.com

'Written by a counselor with years of experience, this book is an exceptional guide for both individuals with traumatic brain injury (TBI) and their families.'
   –**Surendra Barshikar**, MD, MBA, Associate Professor, Vice Chair of Clinical Operations, Medical Director UTSW PMR Clinics, Department of Physical Medicine and Rehabilitation

'Through personal correspondence with survivors and caregivers, Adams explores the complexities of grief, ambiguous loss, and the emotional messiness of recovery, while providing strategies like journaling, prayer, practicing gratitude, and seeking support from others to find a way forward.'
   –**Randi Dubiel**, D.O., Board Certified Physician in Physical Medicine & Rehabilitation and Brain Injury Medicine, Baylor Scott & White Institute for Rehabilitation

'This book is essential for anyone affected by brain injury.'
   –**Amanda Cambra**, LCSW, CBIS, AVP Business Development, Centre for Neuroskills

Letters of Hope and Wisdom for Brain Injury Survivors
Thoughts from a Counselor

Deana Adams

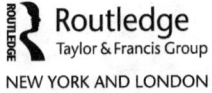
NEW YORK AND LONDON

Designed cover image: getty images via Igor Kutyaev

First published 2026
by Routledge
605 Third Avenue, New York, NY 10158

and by Routledge
4 Park Square, Milton Park, Abingdon, Oxon OX14 4RN

Routledge is an imprint of the Taylor & Francis Group, an informa business

© 2026 Deana Adams

The right of Deana Adams to be identified as author of this work has been asserted in accordance with sections 77 and 78 of the Copyright, Designs and Patents Act 1988.

All rights reserved. No part of this book may be reprinted or reproduced or utilised in any form or by any electronic, mechanical, or other means, now known or hereafter invented, including photocopying and recording, or in any information storage or retrieval system, without permission in writing from the publishers.

Trademark notice: Product or corporate names may be trademarks or registered trademarks, and are used only for identification and explanation without intent to infringe.

Library of Congress Cataloging-in-Publication Data
A catalog record for this title has been requested

ISBN: 978-1-032-99175-7 (hbk)
ISBN: 978-1-032-99174-0 (pbk)
ISBN: 978-1-003-60277-4 (ebk)

DOI: 10.4324/9781003602774

Typeset in Times New Roman
by Taylor & Francis Books

To the thrivers on the brain injury journey

Contents

Foreword ix
Preface xi
Acknowledgements xiii

1 What is Brain Injury? 1
2 Deficits Associated with Brain Injury 12
3 Family Experience of a Loved One with Brain Injury 31
4 Coping with Anxiety 45
5 Coping with Depression 55
6 Coping with Anger 64
7 Relationships 74
8 Grief and Ambiguous Loss 88
9 Trauma and Stress 99
10 Fatigue and Rest 112
11 Events and Holidays 125
12 Self-Esteem and Purpose 135

Appendix A: Visualization – Cloud 149

Appendix B: Outside, Inside 151

Appendix C: Brain Injury Survivor Poem 152

References 154

Index 156

Foreword

The brain has always been my primary area of fascination as a practicing physician (a physiatrist specializing in physical medicine and rehabilitation). It seems that every week, we are learning new and wonderful aspects of how the brain works and interacts with the rest of the body and the world around us. Traumatic injuries to the brain disturb its finely tuned workings. But I have found, over 40 years of caring for people with traumatic brain injuries, that every recovery and every pathway is different, reflecting who each person was before their injury and the particular universe of support and challenge that exists for them. Each is their own person, not just a person with a brain injury.

Sometimes you get lucky with the people you meet along your professional pathway. I have been very lucky to get to know and work with Dr. Deana Adams, a PhD professional counselor with a vast experience in traumatic brain injury, during my time at the University of Texas Southwestern in Dallas. We are pretty different people – Deana from the South, me from the North; Deana a devoted Christian, me a Jew. But our different trajectories brought us to the same place with the same commitment to supporting those with traumatic brain injury in becoming their best selves and recovering a life of dignity and joy. And working with Dr. Adams on education, community support, and individual patients has truly elevated my work as a brain injury physiatrist.

Dr. Adams has a depth of experience as a professional, as a community member, and as a friend in understanding the many outcomes of brain injury. As she describes in this book, there are many medical and cognitive facts to know about recovery from traumatic brain injury. But there are also personal, family, community, and spiritual outcomes that are just as important to talk about and understand.

As I have said, everyone will have a different brain injury and a different path for recovery although many aspects will be shared with other survivors. Because this book is aimed squarely at survivors and their circle of supporters and friends and imbued with the wisdom of Dr. Adams, her many patients, and their care partners, you will undoubtedly find an "a-ha moment" that will speak directly to you.

While medicine will continue to offer improved remedies for brain injury in the future, I'm not convinced that we will ever outrun the brain's capacity to test us. This wisdom and knowledge in this book will be valuable over time regardless of discoveries and treatments.

Kathleen R. Bell, MD
Adjunct Professor
Department of Physical Medicine and Rehabilitation
University of Texas Southwestern
Dallas, Texas
January 7, 2025

Preface

Deana Adams

Today, we are in a winter storm warning here in Texas. That means that everyone hunkers down until the storm passes. It means that we simply do what is necessary to stay warm and nourished. It also means that we are given time to recover and reflect. No one is expecting anything from us. When the elements dictate our behavior and actions, we are obliged to listen. And so it is with brain injury. It is a storm of huge proportions that completely halts the trajectory of life. It changes the individual and family. It causes us to go into crisis mode. Then, after a while, recovery mode. And then, reentry mode. As Dr. Bell mentioned in her Foreword, every person is different. Every brain injury is different.

I'm sitting in my office reflecting about the wonderful people I've met as a professional counselor. I've never been one to shy away from hard things. In fact, I lean into them. Working with brain injury survivors and their families means getting to know close-up both the most difficult and most rewarding population. I love them. They are my heart. I admire how hard they try to learn to live again. I am wowed by their resilience and desire to give back to the community. I am amazed at how well they recover. When I first started working with this population in 2008, counseling did not seem to be on the radar as a viable therapeutic recommendation. I'm happy to report that today, this is not the case.

With every brain injury survivor, I give them the option of having me send them a summary email of our session. Because short-term memory loss is a major issue, I want them to have the email as a reminder. About half of my clients have agreed to receive the emails. It has become an extension of our time together and, frankly, a joy to be able to communicate in written form. I have kept all these emails and correspondence through the years. This book is a compilation of those letters. With all personal information removed, I have separated the emails according to subject matter. Written in layman's terms, each chapter has an educational section and a letter section.

Part 1 is the overview of the effects of brain injury. In the first three chapters, we discuss the effects of a brain injury, what the deficits are, and what experience the family has once a loved one is diagnosed with a brain injury. Part 2 addresses the emotional effects of brain injury. Chapters 4–6 focus on anxiety, depression, and anger. These are the most common emotional issues that occur with survivors and their families. Part 3 focuses on reintegration into the community. Chapters 7–12 address the various issues that are significant in making the transition back to life successful. Learning to be in relationship with others be it friends, family, or acquaintances is addressed in chapter 7. Chapter 8 tackles grief and ambiguous loss. Sometimes survivors experience the death of a friend or loved one in their injury experience. Grieving that loss is part of the healing process. However, the ambiguous losses are numerous. These are abstract losses such as loss of independence, loss of routine, or loss of abilities. Chapter 9 addresses the various traumas and stressors involved in brain injury and its recovery. Chapter 10 explains the need for rest and how to manage fatigue. Chapter 11 gives the reader specific strategies to utilize during holidays and events. The last chapter, Chapter 12, addresses the very important topics of self-esteem and purpose. Although brain injury affects almost all aspects of life, it does not and cannot affect one's spirit. Your brain is injured but your spirit is not. Tapping into the spiritual aspect of life can provide the extra strength and guidance needed to successfully recover from brain injury.

Acknowledgements

Deana Adams

Since 2008 I have had the honor of working with brain injury survivors and their families. Since 2011 I have been the president/founder of Hope After Brain Injury, the only faith-based nonprofit organization for brain injury in the United States. Both venues have offered me a depth of understanding of the world of brain injury. Patti Foster introduced me to traumatic brain injury (TBI) through her own experience. She has welcomed the opportunity to teach me and so many others what it looks like to thrive after a brain injury. Her faith, personality, and indefatigable spirit encourage fellow warriors to keep going and to never give up. You will find more of her story throughout this book. She generously offered her expertise in reviewing the information presented here. I will always be grateful for her dedication and her friendship.

Dr. Kathleen Bell is a one-of-a-kind physician. Not only is she brilliant in her field, but she is also kind in her manner. As a colleague, I've been impressed at her ability to break down complicated medical terms into understandable language for her patients. She introduces herself in the Foreword. You will find a genuine soul. I thank her for joining me and Hope After Brain Injury as we host our annual conferences. Her partnership and friendship enrich my life and my work with brain injury. She graciously reviewed chapter 1, giving me suggestions and corrections to improve and clarify the content. Thank you, Kathy!

Last week after a family session with a TBI survivor and his wife, I was filled with emotion. I sat down and prayed for that family. I prayed for guidance and comfort, for hope and purpose. I prayed that God would make Himself known to this family and meet their needs. I reflected as they represent so many of the brain injury survivors and families that I have known. Each has their own set of challenges that are unique yet similar. I've mentioned some of these friends in the book but have changed their names to protect them. You have my highest admiration.

Early on in my work with brain injury, I met a lady through a chat room. (This was before social media groups.) She had written a poem about her experience as a TBI survivor. Since that time I have shared her poem with thousands of people who have found that it says exactly how they feel. Thank you, Jan, for your vulnerability, for your clear picture of what it's like to live with a brain injury. Her poem, "Outside, Inside", is located in appendix B.

For the Routledge family. Your genuine support and rich enthusiasm have buoyed me in this latest work. Huge thanks go to Lucy Kennedy and Simran Kaur for their kind partnership.

To those of you reading this. I pray that you find wisdom and encouragement. I hope that you feel seen and heard. I trust that you will find some nuggets of truth and strategies to help you cope. Please remember that your recovery is lifelong. There is no stopping point and that is great news! And although we will likely never meet, please know that you have a counselor in Texas cheering you on!

Deana Adams

1 What is Brain Injury?

The Brain

The human brain is a jelly-like substance that sits inside the skull wrapped in three layers of skin-like membrane (meninges). These membranes resemble leather in touch and sight. The inside of the skull is not smooth but rather has bony bumps and ridges that can damage the brain. The brain can move inside the skull if outside forces are applied (like hitting the ground or being thrown back and forth in a car crash). The brain is a complex organ that controls all functions of the human being. At approximately three pounds, this structure is the seat of intelligence, mood, movement, senses, behavior, and every aspect that regulates the body. It is not a muscle but rather an organ that is about 60 percent fat. Forty percent of the brain contains water, protein, carbohydrates, and salts. It contains neurons and blood vessels. The neurons (approximately 100 billion of them) transmit chemical and electrical signals throughout the body sort of like a complex transit system.

Although the full extent of brain activity remains a mystery, we do know about several parts of the brain. The central nervous system is comprised of the brain and spinal cord. The brain stem connects to the spinal cord. During the evolution of the brain, it grows and develops from the back to the front. So, the brain stem (looks like a stalk) controls basic living functions such as breathing, blood pressure, and body temperature. The cerebral cortex is the largest part of the brain and consists of four lobes: occipital, parietal, temporal, and frontal. Functions of these four lobes are generally given below. However, some of the distinct jobs are specific to the right or left hemisphere. The "little brain" called the cerebellum sits above the brain stem and below the occipital and temporal lobes. The two hemispheres of the brain are called the cerebrum and are connected by

DOI: 10.4324/9781003602774-1

a thick bundle of more than 200 million myelinated nerves called the corpus callosum. Myelin is a white, fatty protein substance on the nerve that accelerates electrical impulses and protects the nerve fibers. Deeper structures in the brain include the hypothalamus, thalamus, amygdala, pituitary gland, hippocampus, pineal gland, medulla oblongata, and pons.

Let me highlight some of the functions of each part of the brain mentioned above.

Cerebellum

The cerebellum is a major structure of the hindbrain and holds more than half of the neurons in the body. It plays a role in emotions, voluntary motor skills, and how we make decisions. The cerebellum influences emotional regulation and memory. It can also play a role in inhibiting impulsive behavior. Here are some other functions:

- Balance.
- Movement coordination.
- Posture.
- Visual coordination.
- Mental function of processing language and mood.
- Motor learning like learning to walk or throw a ball.

Occipital Lobe

The occipital lobe sits above the cerebellum and is considered the visual processing center of the brain. It is the smallest lobe of the brain, takes signals from the eyes, and communicates with the rest of the brain. Here are some of the major functions of the occipital lobe:

- Spatial processing: recognizes shapes, textures, and other details of objects.
- Color processing: deciphers the difference between colors and shades of colors.
- Distance and depth perception: calculates size of objects and distance between objects.
- Object and facial recognition: recognizes people and things known prior.
- Information sharing: takes visual information and shares it with other brain areas; helps form memory.

Temporal Lobe

The temporal lobe is located behind the ears, beside the occipital lobe and below the parietal lobe. It is the second-largest lobe in the brain. The two main functions are to process auditory information and encoding of memory. Here are some of the other functions of the temporal lobe:

- Managing your emotions.
- Processing information from your senses.
- Storing and retrieving memories.
- Understanding language (sometimes more than one in different areas).
- Visual recognition of familiar faces and objects.

Parietal Lobe

The parietal lobe sits below your skull at the top rear part of your head between the temporal lobe and frontal lobe. It is the main area that helps you understand where you are in relation to what is happening around you. Here are some of the other functions of the parietal lobe:

- Self-perception: knowing where parts of your body are without looking.
- Location awareness: recognizing left and right.
- Facilitating the performance of learned movements: planning and performing complex movements such as writing.
- Reading.
- Mathematics.

Frontal Lobe

The frontal lobe is in the front portion of the brain and is the largest of the lobes. It is the heart of one's personality and higher functioning and thinking processes. Social skills and managing emotions originate in this area. The frontal lobe continues to mature in individuals until their mid-to-late twenties. The front part of this lobe is called the pre-frontal cortex, which plays a role in memory, judgement, and attention. Here are some other functions of the frontal lobe:

- Abstract thought.
- Creativity.

What is Brain Injury?

- Social appropriateness.
- Executive function such as planning, organizing, and making decisions.
- Paying attention to more than one thing at a time or being able to sustain attention on a single task.
- Linking thoughts to language production or putting thoughts to words.
- Categorizing and comparing objects.
- Assisting in the formation of long-term memory.

The following brain structures are small areas located deep inside the brain.

Hypothalamus

Considered the "smart control" part of the brain, the hypothalamus keeps the body in a balanced state called homeostasis. It manages hormones and your autonomic nervous system (parts of your body that work automatically such as heart rate and breathing). It helps produce hormones (chemical messengers) that regulate your heart rate, sleep/awake cycle, and body temperature. The hypothalamus also helps manage:

- Sex drive.
- Blood pressure.
- Hunger and thirst.
- Sense of fullness when eating.

Thalamus

The thalamus is considered the "train station" because it is the main relay system of the brain. It is an egg-shaped structure in the middle of the brain. One of the main jobs is taking incoming motor and sensory (except smell) information from the body and relaying it to the brain. Here are a few other functions of the thalamus:

- Prioritizes attention by helping choose what to focus on among the vast amount of incoming sensory information.
- Helps process and manage emotion.
- Regulates consciousness (sleep/awake cycle).
- Helps with formation and storage of memory.

Amygdala

The amygdala is an almond-shaped structure within the limbic system (a primitive portion that regulates survival instincts such as hunger, motivation, sex drive, and pain) of the brain (in the temporal lobe). It is the key center for processing emotions such as fear, pleasure, anger, and anxiety. Considered our 24-hour security guard, the amygdala is always aware of environmental stimuli that could be dangerous. It's the part that awakens you when you hear a sound in the night. If you jump when startled, the amygdala is at work! The amygdala attaches emotional content to memories. Interestingly, it is a key structure for forming new memories attached to fear. Here are some other functions of the amygdala:

- Regulates anxiety, aggression, and fear.
- Stores memory.
- Activates the "fight or flight" response.
- Helps recognize emotional responses in facial expressions.

Pituitary Gland

The pituitary gland is the size of a pea and weighs less than a paperclip. It affects your thyroid, adrenal glands, and reproductive system. It is considered the body's "thermostat" because it sends messages in the form of hormones through the organs and glands telling them what is needed and when. It also helps the body and brain respond to stress and trauma. Here are other functions of the pituitary gland:

- Producing a hormone that is essential for labor and lactation.
- Maintaining water and sodium (salt) balance.
- Excreting hormones needed for normal growth and metabolism.

Hippocampus

The hippocampus has a shape like a seahorse and is considered the memory factory of the brain. This small structure located in the temporal lobe has a big job. It helps with memory and learning! Here are specifics about its function:

- Converts short-term memory into long-term memory.
- Helps you remember what words to say (verbal memory).
- Makes you aware of your environment (spatial memory).
- Organizes, retrieves, and stores memory.
- Helps you recall facts (declarative memory).

Pineal Gland

Shaped like a pinecone, the pineal gland is the least-understood and last-discovered part of the endocrine system. Its main job is to help control the circadian rhythm of sleep and wakefulness. This is done by secreting a sleep hormone, melatonin. The French philosopher Descartes believed that the pineal gland was the location of the soul.

Medulla Oblongata

The medulla oblongata is a part of the brain stem connecting the spinal cord to the brain. It is considered a major player in the nervous system because of its location and function. The medulla is involved with partially controlling your heart rate, circulation, and breathing as well as automatic processes like sneezing, coughing, swallowing, and vomiting. It also houses 4 of the 12 cranial nerves that connect from the brain to the body. An interesting characteristic is that the medulla oblongata houses the region of the brain where many of the brain's movement-related neurons "crisscross". The crossover is why one side of the brain controls the opposite side of the body.

Pons

Located just above the medulla oblongata in the brain stem, the pons is a key merging point of several of your cranial nerves. It influences your sleep cycle, manages pain signals, and works with other brain structures to help with balance and movement. Shaped like the top of a cauliflower stalk, the pons helps control pain and movement, particularly in your face and mouth.

Brain Injury

Acquired Brain Injury (ABI) is the umbrella term for all brain injuries. The two main categories of ABI are traumatic brain injury (TBI) and non-traumatic brain injury (NTBI). These are events that happen after birth. ABI is not considered congenital or inherited and is not a result of progressive diseases, like multiple sclerosis. It is considered a leading cause of death and disability worldwide. Simply, traumatic brain injury is damage to the brain that results from an external force and non-traumatic brain injury occurs from an internal source.

NTBI is a brain injury that affects the brain's neuronal activity (nerve signals), physical integrity, and metabolic activity, and the functional ability of the nerves. Examples are strokes, seizures, anoxia (no oxygen), hypoxia (little oxygen), aneurysms, substance abuse, tumors, and infectious diseases such as meningitis or encephalitis. Depending on the research, it has been found that NTBI results in more co-occurring physical health conditions than TBI.

TBI occurs when the brain is damaged due to a strike from the outside of the body such as a forceful bump, blow, or jolt to the head or the body, or even a force that doesn't actually touch the head (as in a high-speed car crash when the brain moves inside the skull, colliding with the bone). Globally, TBI is estimated to affect 27–69 million people annually. TBI is categorized by levels: mild, moderate, severe, and catastrophic. These levels are scored by the Glasgow Coma Scale using three categories: eye response (how well your eyes/pupils respond to stimulus), motor response (how well you can control movement), and verbal response (how well you can answer questions). It is a 15-point test that assesses the severity of brain injury. The higher the number, the less severe. Another predictor of TBI severity is for how long, if at all, there is a loss of consciousness. Mild TBI, commonly known as concussion, accounts for approximately 75 percent of brain injuries. These folks have either no loss or less than 30 minutes' loss of consciousness. Most of the time, people with a single concussion recover completely. However, there are some who continue to have symptoms three months after the initial injury. In this case, the person may be diagnosed with post-concussion syndrome (PCS). Moderate TBI is when there is a loss of consciousness for over 30 minutes but less than 24 hours. Severe TBI is a loss of consciousness for longer than 24 hours. Catastrophic TBI is a loss of all brain function above the brain stem. Memory loss is another factor that determines severity. Not being able to remember events after the injury is called post-traumatic amnesia. The longer the memory loss, the more severe the brain injury. The range is less than 24 hours to longer than 4 weeks. Retrograde amnesia is the inability to remember events prior to the injury. This indicates a more severe brain injury. None of these predictors are 100% reliable. Some people with very severe TBI make unexpected amounts of recovery. Research is now examining other ways of determining preserved brain function using advanced imaging; this is still happening at a research level.

There are two basic types of TBI: penetrating and non-penetrating. As the name indicates, penetrating TBI is when the skull is pierced and something enters the brain tissue such as a bullet, shrapnel, or bone fragments. Non-penetrating is also considered blunt force trauma or closed head injury and may result in a localized area of bleeding in or around the brain. Diffuse axonal injury (DAI) also falls under non-penetrating injury. This is when the brain itself moves inside the skull with such force that the nerves are sheared in a characteristic pattern.

What are the causes of TBI? Depending on several factors such as age, gender, parts of the country, and parts of the world, these causes differ in prevalence. Generally, around the world, falls are considered the most common. Other causes are motor vehicle crashes, sports injuries, assaults, blast injuries, intimate partner violence, and being struck from or by an object such as bumping your head against a door. In one given event such as a car wreck, a person can experience both a non-penetrating and a penetrating injury. For example, a driver is hit from behind by someone going over the speed limit. The initial brain injury could be the jolt of the vehicle being hit. The person could also be ejected out of the car, thereby being struck by flying debris, and have a penetrating head injury.

It's important to recognize that all of us start out with strengths and weaknesses in terms of our abilities. That's one of the reasons it is so hard to predict how people will recover afterwards – we are all wired differently although, in general, our brains are designed in the same patterns.

Let's talk about the brain and the injury from the counselor's office.

Letter to You

Dear Friend,

You may have heard me say this before but let me tell you again. You are a hero! I cannot think of anyone who embodies resilience as well as you do. In fact, you are twice as smart as the rest of us! Why? Because you learned to live. You had the injury. And now you are learning to live again. That's twice as smart! You are this world's best-kept secret of how to live courageously and valiantly. I want to do all I can to encourage and infuse you with hope that you can become the person you are meant to be. Brain injury happened to you. It does not define you. It is a part of your story, not your whole story. Yes, your life has changed. Only you can determine whether for the best or worse. Tragedy can strengthen us in the end. Just like Jesus showed his scars to his disciple, Thomas (who doubted Jesus' death and resurrection in John 20:27–31), so you can show people your scars. They tell a story. Let yours be a story of overcoming. Tara was in a car wreck on her way to work. She was hit by a truck hauling a tractor. When asked about her facial lacerations and subsequent scars, she said with gentle pride, "I want people to see my scars. They tell a story. I earned them."

Even though we hear about it more often nowadays, brain injury is still a mystery to most people. I imagine that you feel alone. That makes sense. It's hard to feel connected to others when most of your friends and family know little to nothing about TBI. It's almost like you have to educate them. In one way, that is good. In another, it's super-hard because it can take a lot out of you. And because the brain is so complex, no two brain injuries are alike. You may have heard the saying, "If you've seen one brain injury, you've seen one brain injury." That is so true! On one hand you want people to get it, on the other you don't want them to have to go through brain injury in order to get it. Let me encourage you to connect with a support group of TBI survivors in your area. The family also needs support from other caregivers. This is a long road so why not have some companions who have already walked it? The two greatest needs for those on the brain injury journey are patience and understanding. Having a peer that gets it can provide both. If you need help finding a support group, ask your local rehabilitation hospital. They typically know the current groups. Plus, don't hesitate to look online. There are quite a few online support groups. Be mindful of seeking groups that are positive and who offer suggestions and help. Healthy groups are not negatively focused. If you have been online with someone in a group and you feel better afterwards, it is likely that you are in a healthy group. If you feel worse, it is probably not a good fit.

One of the scriptures that reminds me of the extravagant brain is Psalm 139:14 (New International Version) which says in part "I am fearfully and wonderfully made." You are! And guess what? You were born with several million extra brain cells! So, you already had brain cells ready to work when your brain injury happened. Someone once explained it like this: when a brain injury happens, it is like the telephone wires of the brain fell and snapped. The gift of neuroplasticity (nerve cells are created and strengthened) helps gain some of what was lost in the injury. It is the process of reconnecting or recreating those telephone wires. And you know, we only know so much about the brain. Thankfully, more is being discovered each day.

Do your best to draw on your faith. Whether you are Muslim, Jewish, Hindu, Protestant, Catholic, or Pagan, allow the faith community to support you and walk alongside you. Positive religious coping helps you gain strength and direction from one's Higher Power. Allow your TBI to draw you closer to your faith. Prayer and meditation are two ways that can improve one's state of mind. Mindfulness is another way that helps you focus on the here and now. These exercises help you focus on the spiritual aspect of recovery. Use your spirituality as a resource towards healing.

As much as you can, complete each stage of recovery. Even though the multiple doctor visits and therapy visits can be exhausting, please take advantage of them. It's OK, though, to take a break every now and then. I call it "therapy fatigue". Let your providers know that you will take a week off to recuperate. Rest, but don't quit. It is common for survivors to want to leave the treatment before they are discharged. Part of that is because they do not have the awareness of the impact of the injury. Another part is because therapy is hard and taxing. You may notice that for every one appointment you need one day of rest. One friend said that she must schedule three days of rest for one social event. Another friend said that if he has two therapy appointments in one day, he takes the weekend off to rest. Your pace may be different. Honor what your brain and body need. Do your best not to push yourself to do more than you should. That creates more mistakes and setbacks. A slower pace is more effective. Like I often say, "Add grace to your pace." Be kind to yourself and allow for the downtime. It will go a long way in helping you recover.

Finally, I want you to know that you are on the frontier of brain injury recovery. Even though most people are familiar with the term "traumatic brain injury", the field is still new. Your success will help other survivors down the road. No tragedy is without redemption. Your pain can comfort someone else. Be encouraged to know that where you are today is not where you will be tomorrow. Brain injury is a bit inconsistent from day to day but overall, it is a slow progression. As long as you have breath, you have the opportunity to grow and improve and recover. We have friends in our support group 60-plus years in recovery and still finding areas of improvement. You can too. It's never too late.

With huge respect,
Deana

Homework

- Each day write two positives and one challenge. For example, two positives would be: I made cereal. I got dressed. The challenge would be: I got too tired.

What is Brain Injury?

- Share with your caregiver one thing s/he did that was helpful to you. (Sometimes we forget to be grateful for the help!)

_____

_____

Resources

Keep this heading and remove references

References

Gronwall, D., Wrightson, P., & Waddel, P. (1998). *Head injury: The facts.* (2nd ed.). Oxford University Press.

Adler, R. (2021). *Understanding traumatic brain injury: A guide for survivors and families.* Word Association Publishers.

2 Deficits Associated with Brain Injury

Now that you have an idea about the brain and how it functions, let's look at some of the deficits of a brain injury. The word "deficit" means a lack of function or an impairment in functional capacity. In other words, deficit is a result of the brain injury itself. Because every brain is different and every brain injury is different, this description and discussion about deficits is generalized. A wonderful aspect of deficits is that they do change. Think about a deficit as a continuum, meaning there is a variation of degrees from severe to mild. Maybe in the beginning stages of TBI, the deficits are more pronounced or evident. In the later stages of recovery, some of the deficits can be just as obvious and others are less obvious. Unfortunately, there is no clear-cut picture of your specific brain injury. So, let me share with you a general view of deficits commonly linked to certain areas of the brain.

Deficits

Short-Term Memory Loss

Memory is stored in various locations throughout the brain. For example, the hippocampus and amygdala store explicit memory (memory from specific events throughout our lives). Implicit memory (like motor memory) is stored in the basal ganglia and cerebellum. For example, riding a bike is a motor memory that is accessed from that location. Working memory (comprehension, problem-solving, reasoning, learning) comes from the prefrontal cortex, the frontmost part of the brain's frontal lobe. This is the part of the memory that helps one complete tasks. Although working memory is associated with short-term memory (STM), it retains information a bit longer than STM. The hippocampus, located inside the temporal lobe, is one of the main areas that stores STM. This is memory that lasts for a few seconds.

DOI: 10.4324/9781003602774-2

Normally, STM is associated with simple tasks or recent events, small bits of information in a short amount of time.

The most common type of memory loss after a TBI is short-term memory loss. Some of the ways that STM loss presents are:

- Not remembering a task or event. For example, going to the store but forgetting what to buy or not remembering what you had for breakfast.
- Problems with multitasking and/or doing two things at once. This may include forgetting to complete the laundry because you forgot the clothes were in the washer. Or turning on the TV and forgetting that you have food in the microwave.
- Not being able to find the right words to use. This also means using the wrong word.
- Not remembering details about a conversation.
- Forgetting the day or time of day.
- Not remembering what was watched on television or read in a book.
- Not remembering appointments or medication.

Thankfully, there are wonderful coping strategies to help with STM loss. You may have a few of your own. Generally, the skills listed below are helpful:

1. Eliminate distractions. It is important to concentrate on the topic at hand in order to remember or write down the task. Eliminating extra noise, conversation, or multiple sensory demands will help the survivor concentrate.
2. Have a memory notebook. This is the "go-to" book where you write down chores, appointments, names of people, etc. Amy Grant, the gospel singer, experienced a TBI from a bicycle accident. She had several notebooks that kept the words of her songs, the important people in her life, and her schedule. You may create your own system. Many survivors also use the note section on their mobile device. Others use a paper calendar to jot down events or things to remember.
3. Use a pill box to keep your medicine organized.
4. Use a whiteboard. These are great visual reminders of events, appointments, and things to do. It is recommended to hang the whiteboard in a high-traffic area in the home such as the kitchen.
5. Keep things to remember in one place. For example, the car keys are always placed on the counter. Or the cell phone is stored at the charging station.

6 Repeat information as needed.
7 Use an alarm clock to help remember when to take medication or other things that you do not want to forget. Often, cell phones have an alarm, which works well to remind the person of certain things.
8 Make lists. Whether one has a brain injury or not, lists help keep one organized.
9 Practice remembering names. This is to help strengthen the memory factories in the brain.
10 Break down chores into small steps. This helps keep the survivor from feeling overwhelmed and possibly forgetting some of the steps.
11 Create routine. For example, go to bed and get up at the same times each day.
12 Do one thing at a time.

Hopefully, some of these strategies will help strengthen your brain and improve your memory.

Flooding

Flooding is when the senses are overwhelmed. It happens because the brain's filter system is damaged. Some of our TBI friends describe it as "my filter system is gone" or "I don't have a filter." In other words, your brain cannot filter out unwanted sounds or sights. Environmental stimuli come into the brain all with the same magnitude and intensity. The brain cannot filter background noise or indirect lighting as a passive stimulus. It is all processed to the same degree. When the brain is flooded, it can "freeze", making it difficult to maintain a conversation or be in a room. Some survivors describe flooding as brain overload, or their wits are overwhelmed. Sensory overload symptoms include agitation, anxiety, difficulty breathing, or fatigue. Some of the triggers of flooding are:

- Noise such as radio, television, or loud conversation.
- Sight such as multicolored signs, flashing lights, or complicated patterns.
- Unpleasant tastes.
- Unexpected movement such as rocking, being shoved, or being touched abruptly.
- Smells such as cleaning solution, candles, or strong odors.
- Electronic devices such as cell phones, computers, or laptops.

Managing a flooding episode starts with recognizing what triggers you. Consider making a list of things that tend to overwhelm you or triggers that set you off or make you uncomfortable. Then, create a list of ways to manage the event. For example, at night, asking loved ones to turn off or put away electronic devices to avoid light rays and noise that keep one from good rest and sleep. At the event, when the band is playing too loud, give yourself permission to find a quiet room. If going to church feels overwhelming, consider asking your loved one to let you sit at the end of a row so you can leave when needed. Wearing a ball cap or hat and sunglasses will help reduce the visual stimuli. Also, wearing earplugs mutes some of the noise. These helps can make it easier for you to participate in an event. One of our TBI friends says that going to her granddaughter's recitals is very difficult for her because of all the noise, cross talk, people, and general excitement about the events. So she wears sunglasses, double earplugs, and a hat. She also brings a hand fan to use if she feels too hot. She said that the accessories helped her attend the events. She also schedules a rest day after each recital to recover and recuperate. We will talk more about how to manage events in chapter 11.

Challenges with Academic Skills

Sometimes with a brain injury, survivors have trouble with writing, math, reading, or comprehension. The loss of academic skills often makes the survivor feel stupid or less smart. This is a good time to remind them that their brain is healing and that these skills will come back. Brain injury is brain injury, not a loss of intelligence. Academic challenges, in part, are due to damage to the parietal lobe of the brain. Depending on the severity of the brain injury, academic skills deficits may differ in their severity. Interestingly, many of the TBI survivors with whom I work struggle with basic math. One of my friends graduated with two master's degrees from MIT (Massachusetts Institute of Technology) yet could not balance his checkbook after his automobile accident. Another friend was an accountant with an international finance company and struggled to input data in an Excel sheet. Eventually, he was able to return to his accounting position and perform well. The card game Uno is used by many rehabilitation centers to help survivors with numbers, counting, and problem-solving.

Reading is also a challenge. Having to relearn the alphabet and understanding syllables and consonants are all difficult when the brain has been damaged. If there are accompanying vision problems, reading from the left to the right is challenging. If one has dizziness, the eye movement can cause nausea. Comprehending the words in a sentence is a slower process than before the injury. As mentioned above, recalling the context or details of what was previously read can be a challenge so that you may need to reread the same passage over again. One of our survivor friends joked that she never has to buy new books because she just rereads the ones she has.

Writing takes coordination and fine motor skills. With a brain injury, these abilities can be limited or slowed or missing altogether. Many times, they must be relearned. Using a computer keyboard requires similar skills along with processing challenges. The good news is that most survivors can recover these skills with time and practice. Learning to write your name can be helpful in developing writing skills. Interestingly, this "simple" practice tends to take a lot of cognitive energy. One of my TBI friends struggles with writing her name. Not that she doesn't know how, but because it "wears her out". She becomes fatigued.

Depending on the severity of the brain injury and depending on what part of the brain has been impacted, most of the academic skills can be regained. It takes patience, practice, and encouragement. As one of our friends suggests, celebrate every small step of recovery.

Mood Swings

Mood swings that accompany brain injury are not the same as mood swings of bipolar disorder. Generally, mood swings due to bipolar disorder are depressive episodes and mania episodes that last several weeks each. In other words, someone struggling with the mental illness will feel depressed for weeks to months. Then, they will feel "high" or "manic" for weeks or months. Mood swings for survivors are caused by damage to the areas of the brain that control emotions and behavior. They are referred to as mood swings because the survivor may be laughing and a short time later (sometimes in the same conversation) the survivor is sad and crying. Just as quickly, agitation and anger may flare. It can be very confusing for both the survivor and the care partner. It is best to observe, not judge or take the emotional changes personally. Let it be information for you. What contributes to the confusion is that the emotional response may not be what the survivor is feeling. One of our survivor friends will laugh when she is upset about something. She is not happy, but her brain is making her laugh. Some may cry but do not feel sad. Often the emotional changes are a stage in the early parts of recovery. When there is an emotional reaction, give the survivor time and a quiet space to calm down and regain control. Acknowledge that there is a feeling about something. Then, gently and kindly help the survivor talk about the feeling. Talking about it helps both the survivor and family member gain a better understanding of what may have caused the emotional reaction. It also gives an opportunity to develop a game plan if it should happen in the future. It may also be that the survivor has a hard time verbalizing or talking about what happened. Do your best not to step on their silence but give them space to formulate and speak their thoughts. A survivor recommended the listener to not try to guide or guess what the survivor is trying to say. This is an opportunity to practice trying to understand the survivor and be patient with him.

Lack of Awareness and Impulsivity

The lack of awareness is a result of injury to the frontal lobe as well as the parietal lobe. The technical term for this condition is anosognosia. Very basically, the survivor does not acknowledge that he has any deficits. Physical issues are seen and considered. But issues on an emotional or cognitive level simply do not exist to the survivor. Not having insight into one's impairment can be complicated for the family. Mostly because the family recognizes the limitations, but the survivor tends to deny it. The denial is not because the survivor wants to be difficult but rather, he does not recognize deficits. This is one reason why it is important for the counselor to get feedback from family members as well as the survivor. Typically, some survivors have impaired reasoning, impulsiveness, attention or concentration problems, and poor compliance to treatment. Sometimes the lack of awareness makes the survivor deny impulsive behavior or recognize that there are consequences to their actions. Additionally, they have a hard time recognizing what another person is feeling. Curtis fell off a ladder at work. Even though he was hospitalized and participated in rehabilitation, he never thought that he had a TBI. In fact, any time his wife mentioned it, he thought she was lying or picking on him. Although he was given full-time nursing assistance to oversee his care, he thought that they were only there to help his wife. The nature of his TBI did not allow him to recognize any deficit or challenge.

Saying or doing things without thinking in advance is called impulsiveness. The technical term for this condition is disinhibition. This is a part of the "lack of awareness" aspect of brain injury. Often it is the result of frontal lobe injury. Impulsivity makes it hard to resist urges or inhibit impulses. Some of the ways that a survivor shows impulsiveness are by interrupting a conversation. Another impulsive act is rushing into a decision without thinking it through. It is as though the survivor reacts first and thinks about the consequences later. Other signs of impulsive behavior are spending all of one's money in a short space of time; getting into relationships too quickly; signing a contract without fully understanding what it means; and having regrets about decisions or statements. Driving too fast or not following the rules are two more examples of impulsiveness.

Coping strategies to manage lack of awareness and impulsiveness include having a limited amount of money to spend. Sometimes external boundaries are needed to keep a loved one from being taken advantage of or impulsively buying something. Consider creating a budget and do your best to stick to it. Self-regulation is a coping skill that takes practice and intention. The survivor may want to ask their family members to help them when they are interrupting a conversation or making a financial decision. I advise my clients to enlist a trusted family member to discuss decisions before committing to something. The survivor may also practice not interrupting, or waiting to ask a trusted loved one before spending money. Sometimes writing notes of what he wants to work on is helpful. Unfortunately, many survivors are taken advantage of because of their impulsiveness and because they tend to believe what is being told to them. So, if a stranger tells them of their woes and that they just need a few dollars, the survivor is likely to give it to them. They have not yet regained the awareness that people can be deceiving. Consider not having an open-door policy to all software and internet activity, meaning: have some protected sites and supervise any comments or posts made to the survivor. One may delete promotional emails, ads, or shopping apps. This is a way to protect your loved one from cyberbullying or scam artists. Another part of self-regulation for the survivor is asking himself questions that will help him make a healthy decision. Keeping these questions in sight or accessible will help the survivor reference them as needed.

These can be questions such as:

- "Do I need this?"
- "What are other options?"
- "What are the pros and cons?"
- "If I do this, what will happen next?"

One of our survivor friends has a note in her office that says "close your mouth" to help remind her to not say whatever comes to mind. If the survivor has realized that he said something rude or tactless, he can apologize. Accepting his apology goes a long way in helping him remedy a situation and create a way to solve problems in the future.

Responding to impulsive behavior in a positive way is more effective than reacting in a negative way. Help direct behavior without taking over and completing the task for him; this helps him gain independence. Kind oversight helps the survivor eventually self-regulate, meaning he can develop the skills needed to behave in a more steady and reasonable manner.

Coordination and Balance

Coordination and balance problems are common after a brain injury. Balance is being able to keep your body centered over your base of support (feet, thighs, butt). There are a couple of main regions in the brain responsible for coordination and balance. The brain stem and the cerebellum control balance, fine and gross motor skills, and coordination. Symptoms of balance issues are dizziness, unsteadiness, or disequilibrium. There are a multitude of reasons that cause balance problems. They could be related to vision impairment, medication, inner ear problems, blood pressure issues, inability to feel things, or brain stem injury. Also, if someone has had an extended hospital stay and has not been able to get out of bed, his strength will have deteriorated. So, it takes time to regain strength. Often, occupational and physical therapy are recommended to help the survivor relearn mobility and function.

It is important to address balance and coordination issues not only to avoid falls but also to maneuver safely throughout the events of the day. Physical therapy works specifically to help with coordination and balance. Occupational therapy helps with fine motor skills along with skills needed to perform activities of daily living. Vestibular therapy focuses on balance and dizziness. It is a type of physical therapy that uses exercises to help the brain, eyes, and body work together. Regular practice of exercises helps improve coordination and increases strength. Adaptive exercises are customized to address physical disabilities or special needs of a person. *Love Your Brain* is an adaptive yoga program created especially for brain injury survivors. Another adaptive exercise is using a recumbent bike to accommodate poor balance or limited mobility such as back or neck issues.

Personality Changes

One of the most challenging aspects of a brain injury is personality change. This is one of the aspects of having an "invisible injury" because the injury is on the inside. It is especially hard when the survivor looks the same as before the injury. Personality originates in several parts of the brain. The frontal, temporal, and parietal lobes contribute to one's personality. Phineas Gage, a railroad worker in the 1800s, experienced a TBI from a work explosion. A large 13-pound tamping iron accidentally exploded, entering his lower jaw and exiting the top of his skull. Mr. Gage's accident was one of the first cases studied that documented a personality change after a brain injury. His personality changed from an even-tempered man to one who was irreverent, ill-tempered, and impatient. Some of the characteristics of someone with brain injury include the tendency to be self-focused, less motivated, less aware of the needs of others, quick to anger, becoming obsessive or inflexible, losing the ability to control emotions, or becoming childlike in manner. Their sense of humor tends to change as well. For example, some survivors do not understand clever or higher-level jokes but show a preference for slapstick humor. Some survivors are less interested in social activity and would rather stay home. This may be in part because of the sensory overload in social settings. Sometimes personality traits become more intense after brain injury. Some traits are less noticeable. For example, Roger became "emotionless" after his brain injury. His pre-injury personality was jovial and entertaining. Now, he says that he does not feel at all. Another survivor reports not being able to cry, when before the injury, she often cried at a sad movie or sad circumstances. Claudia says that she has "more" of a personality. She stated that she is the same person but feels things more deeply and for longer than before the injury. Some survivors use more explicit language or obscenities after a brain injury. This is especially off-putting if someone was mild-mannered before. Because there is a loss of a filter, some survivors will say whatever comes to mind whether it is appropriate or inappropriate. It can be that the survivor is not able to pick up on social cues. This is something he can learn through the various therapies in rehabilitation. Again, these changes are because the brain has been affected, not because the survivor is intentionally being different. As a counselor, it is helpful to remember that the survivor will continue to improve, just not quickly or at a predictable pace.

    Managing personality change can be difficult. It is challenging for the survivor and for the family members. It is helpful to remember that the survivor's personality will continue to evolve as his brain heals. One of the care partners said something that is important regarding personality changes. She said that she tries not to compare her post-injury husband to the pre-injury husband because the two are completely different. She did not believe it was fair to compare him to someone he is not. Another care partner said that she has been married to two men without getting a divorce. Some spouses have difficulty living with someone whom they did not marry. In other words, the person looks the same but the personality is so different. In many cases, the spouse learns to love the new post-injury personality. This was true with one of my friends. During the time between their engagement and wedding, her husband had experienced a TBI. She interpreted his more jovial, less filtered conversations as his excitement to marry. It wasn't until later that she recognized that his personality had changed. They have been intentional about communicating and correcting his behavior in healthy, non-confrontational ways. For example, when he spends too long on a topic of conversation, she will touch his hand. He knows that her touching his hand is a signal between them that he needs to wind down the conversation.

Sometimes the nature of the brain injury causes the survivor to regress emotionally and behaviorally. Janet, an adult TBI survivor, said that she watched children's television with her younger sibling because it was easy and entertaining to her. Chris, the wife of a TBI survivor, said that she has watched her husband grow up from being a toddler emotionally to an adolescent and then to an adult. As mentioned earlier, it is most helpful to observe these behaviors and changes instead of judging them. Just as a normal (non-head-injured) person continues to grow and adapt, the survivor will mature and develop socially, personally, and academically.

Inflexible or Rigid Thinking

A brain injury can cause many cognitive deficits. Inflexible thinking is one of those. This rigid thinking is the inability to switch from one topic to another or from one activity to another. It is also called perseveration. An example of this is when the survivor talks on and on about the same topic. Sometimes he may get stuck on a certain word or phrase or thought. Normally this happens when there is damage to the frontal cortex, which controls self-awareness and self-restraint. The survivor may also stay in an emotion longer than the situation warrants. He may shake hands with someone longer than necessary. Rigid thinking happens when the brain's "telephone wires" haven't reconnected yet. Many of these behaviors are also due to damaged social skills. Part of speech therapy is helping the survivor practice "give and take" in conversation. A trusted loved one is key to helping the survivor practice the social skills and reminding him of social graces and mores.

Strategies to help your loved one who is perseverating include recognizing the behavior. Edward was a historian before his injury. After his injury, he would "get stuck" on the topic of history. So, his wife came up with a "stuck signal" that helped him recognize that he was speaking too long on the topic of history. The survivor may set an alarm to help remind himself to stop talking about a certain subject. As the survivor recovers and neuroplasticity improves the neural pathways, the rigid thinking will lessen. It is important to recognize and praise the survivor when he redirects his behavior or conversation. Again, perseveration will lessen as the brain reconnects or grows new neural pathways in the frontal cortex and parts of the brain that control awareness and discipline.

Letter to You

Dear Friend,

Have I told you that you are twice as smart as the rest of us? Because you learned to live; had a brain injury; and now you are learning to live again! You are an amazing testament to resilience! You have overcome adversity and bounced back despite huge life stressors. Let's talk about some of the deficits of brain injury and how to cope with them. Perhaps some of these insights will bring hope and tools to navigate your daily life with brain injury. I will also share a few insights into managing various life challenges like travel, social events, and general everyday life. Perhaps you have your own strategies to add!

Here are some thoughts about memory, awareness, and processing. Both short-term and long-term memory can be affected by brain injury. It's weird because you may remember something from yesterday and forget what happened 10 minutes ago or vice versa. Short-term memory tends to be an issue with the majority of brain injury survivors. Create your own way to remind yourself of things. For example, one friend would put the laundry basket by her sofa to remind her that clothes were in the washer. Long-term memory either can be spontaneous recall or needs a "hint". Examples of a hint are saying the first letter of a word or "sounds like" or giving the circumstance around the event. Emotional and factual memories are stored in different parts of the brain. Details about the event are held in one part of the brain. How you feel about the event is stored in a different part of the brain. So, that's why you may remember a feeling as opposed to an actual "play-by-play". For example, I don't remember what happened, but I remembered that it was fun (or bad or whatever). Just because you lose a memory, it doesn't mean you are losing your mind. You are not crazy nor are you going crazy. Your brain is injured.

Brain injury recovery never happens lickety-split...you will notice progress in weeks and months, not hours and days. I wanted to point this out because in relationships, it can get difficult when the survivor remembers or forgets randomly. That's just part of the memory storage and retrieval process, not a personality or paying attention/not paying attention issue. With a TBI, slower processing is part and parcel of the injury. Please know that these memory issues can improve over time. Your processor is a bit slower, not your IQ. By the way, do your best to not keep comparing your present self with your pre-injury self.

Fatigue makes the deficits harder to manage. So, please honor your brain's signal to rest. Take a break. Please know that the difficulties with memory are connected to stress as well. What is true is that you are going through "growing pains" cognitively. Another truth is that you are building your brain and improving the neuron connections (nerves are being rerouted or recreated through neuroplasticity) because of all the new things you are having to navigate. So, be encouraged. Your brain is getting stronger; your heart is getting lighter; your stress is getting manageable. You are developing new neuropathways in your brain. It doesn't happen from speed only; it comes with repetition and gentleness. And the recovery is inconsistent. So, practice extending kindness to yourself and your healing timeline. When you are fatigued, take a break. When you are angry, replace it with compassion. In other words, give yourself a place to walk away to and calm down or simply change the subject.

Being aware of the deficits can be a challenge. Sometimes survivors recognize they have a brain injury but are unaware of how it manifests in daily life. For example, one of my TBI friends said that she has trouble in social settings because she is awkward. She has been asked to leave certain social events because she makes rude or insensitive comments. She is aware of the injury, but not aware of how it makes her (and other people) feel. Typically, the less awareness, the more blame. So, if someone gets upset and the survivor does not recognize his role in the problem, he will blame the difficulty on other people or other circumstances. The brain injury does not always recognize when something is insensitive or inappropriate. It is helpful to have a loved one help the survivor recognize issues before they erupt.

Filter absence is a deficit that often comes with most frontal lobe damage. That means you may say things before you realize the impact of them. Eventually, you will be able to create your own filter either through walking away or by biting your tongue. This, too, will get better. The filter system is not working with output or input, meaning there is no filter to catch words from being said and no filter to screen out unnecessary noises or lights. Therefore, please be mindful of "incoming" stimulation such as someone else's anxiety, noise, or complicated visuals. You must be intentional about protecting yourself from external stimulus. It is not something your brain will do on its own as in the past. Don't be shy about finding ways to eliminate the intensity of noise or lights. For example, using lower-wattage light bulbs. The filter now is intentional, not natural.

Flooding happens in part because of the no-filter. It is when there is too much external stimulus for your brain to process. Other words that describe flooding are feeling overwhelmed or bombarded or experiencing a brain surge. You can't help when your brain shuts down and can't think. Really, it's just a sign from you to you to step back and take a break. One trick you may try...shut your eyes for about 10–15 seconds and see if that doesn't help bring your brain back online. The best way to manage an episode is to remove yourself from the stimulus. For example, if the conversation becomes too much to process, excuse yourself for a few minutes and go to a quieter room. Normal people do not realize how much energy it takes you to think, process, decide because it comes naturally to them. However, it's no longer natural for you. Because of that, please do your best to reduce outside stimulation (noise, lights, conversation). If you are required to make a decision, please try to have the conversation away from the stimulus.

Hypersensitivity happens when any external sensory input such as sounds, lights, etc. is felt more strongly than by a normal person. Same thing with words...if someone raises his voice, the survivor is probably going to perceive that in a negative way. Even when it comes to simple frustration about life circumstances, he will take it personally. This is a brain injury thing, not a survivor being too sensitive thing, although it looks the same. Taking things personally is especially present at the early stages of recovery. It will lessen but be a "tender" place further along in the healing process. Basically, he doesn't have a filter for incoming stimulation. That also means it will take him longer to process the incident. So, my thoughts on combating or navigating hypersensitivity are:

1   Use a gentler tone when speaking to your loved one.
2   Picture in your mind that the brain is exposed or an unprotected wound, if you will. This will help you approach the survivor more gently.
3   A survivor's thoughts are super-critical already. I've seen this across the board with brain injury. They tend to second-guess and doubt themselves mercilessly. So, consider a kind approach with correction.

Here are some tips from survivors to other survivors:

- Best time is in the morning so do hard stuff then.
- Journal/write.
- Take vitamins/eat healthy.
- Exercise, preferably outside.
- Encourage others.
- Create your own motto for living.
- Persevere and don't give up.
- Meditation/prayer.
- Eat a popsicle when you have a headache.
- Have mercy on yourself...be kind and compassionate to yourself.
- Hold your tongue (don't lose your temper).

TBI is an unseen injury. The emotional and cognitive challenges are invisible to most people. It's OK and normal to feel frustrated and angry and upset. Sometimes brain injury makes it hard to manage your emotions. It's almost like they are on overdrive or underdrive. Believe it or not, the emotional ups and downs are part of the healing process. Try not to judge it. Do pay attention to the pattern...see if you are able to control your emotions a bit more. As you know, any emotional output, whether happy, sad, or anger, zaps your energy. Please know that as long as you have breath, you have growth with the brain. Please trust that. No, it doesn't move as fast as we would like, but it does move at its own pace.

Use the safe space to heal...find joy, experience peace, cry, grieve... and then have fun. Give yourself a break and play. Then, go back at it. You may have to do that same routine over and over again. The remedy for stress is rest, gratitude, breathe, pace, grace. If you practice one of those coping strategies, you will find that you can manage your stress better. So, rest or take a break. Make a list of what you are thankful for. Breathe deeply and slowly. Do not rush but pace yourself. And, always extend grace (instead of criticism) to yourself by remembering you are doing the best that you can at any given moment.

Also, another challenge is the rigidity that comes with brain injury. The brain needs structure to grow and get better. So, changing plans or having too much flexibility can be counterproductive and lead to outbursts and misunderstandings. A loose schedule is much better than a tight one. Please be kind to yourself. Give yourself grace. Cry when you need to and laugh when you can.

One of my TBI survivors said that she tried to function at "medium-low" level. For her, it was a brilliant coping skill to help her get through each event of the day. She said that this level of energy helped her not get too fatigued too quickly. Additionally, I often tell my survivors to do or schedule only one big thing a day and do one thing at a time. Do not multitask. For example, a therapy appointment will be the one big thing. Rest and do tasks with low cognitive requirements outside of the one big thing. I can only imagine how frustrating it is to not be able to function at your normal high level. I am impressed at your ability to still create. I think that's a huge cognitive process that remains with you. As we discussed, the processor is a bit slow. Pacing is going to be your main coping strategy. That means adding rest periods when available. Re-creating a new life is allowing you and God to co-create. Please think about ways you can reduce your energy output instead of how one can push through. Continue to pace yourself according to your capacity. It's OK to delay certain cognitive assignments. It's OK to delay conversations with certain people. It's OK. Reality is harsh enough. Add gentleness as a significant thread in your new life.

Just a hint about multitasking. At the beginning of your recovery, you can only do one thing at a time. That is OK and expected. However, as you recover you may be able to do two things at the same time such as writing and listening to music. It's not easy to go about doing one thing and get interrupted by a question from someone else. It throws you off and frustrates the questioner. You may want to say "just a minute" or "hold on" when a question gets to you; finish your task; and then follow up with the request. The interruption is never meant to frustrate you, but the extra cognitive skills required to process two things are oftentimes too much. When you are able to do two things at once, count it as a win and as a sign you are getting better. Patti, our TBI survivor friend, suggests writing a note on a sticky pad to help you remember what you are doing. You may write down a word that will give you a hint of what you were doing before you were interrupted.

Just remember, you are getting better because you are realizing what you can do. One of the struggles with TBI is being very sensitive. Your feelings may hurt easily if you perceive someone putting you down or being mean. You may get offended when someone says or does something, even when they didn't mean it offensively. Part of coping with that is you realizing you may be misreading the situation and part of it is the other person being mindful of how they are saying something and how they are coming across. One of the biggest helps when in an argument is to not take things personally. This is a learned response, not natural at all. We, as humans, tend to take things personally. But in brain injury, that makes things worse. So, do your best to not take things personally. Please give each other grace. It's hard to come back to life. Your future can be better than you can imagine. Get to know one another again.

Please be kind to yourself. So, that means, don't be mean to yourself if you miss a social cue or forget something or get talking about a variety of things. Gently lead yourself back to the conversation/topic at hand. Give yourself the option to pivot (change direction or change the plan) when a loved one is requiring more of you, or you are experiencing a difficult day. Pivot to adjust the plan and one's thinking about the plan. There are life experiences that most people don't recognize as difficult…yet they are. Normal people rarely realize that, for a TBI survivor, every action takes thought. Every step takes thought. Every chew/swallow takes thought. So, give yourself space to think and recover…think and recover…think and recover.

Here are some tips on how to manage brain drain:

1 Ask for time and space: tell someone to "hold on a minute" while you finish your thought. This will help take the pressure off answering a question or explaining yourself. Consider "I'll get back to you" as a comment that gives you more time to think about something. Sometimes you may need to just walk away.
2 Manage sensory downloads: use your earplugs or sunglasses, reduce exposure.
3 Require less of yourself: remind yourself that today, I have the capacity to do X. Or, I do not have the capacity to do X. And be OK and gracious with yourself either way. Understanding how much you are able to accomplish in any given time takes experience. At first, you may not recognize how much is too much. Consider smiling or making someone laugh or point out something else to take the pressure off.
4 Schedule rest: giving yourself time to reflect and rest leads to restoration.

5 Creativity: playing the piano or doing something creative tends to give one energy. Plus, it's a great training exercise for cognitive improvement! One of our survivor friends plays frisbee, goes for a walk, and bakes to be creative. The great thing about creativity is that you don't have to go by the rules!
6 Play: includes doing puzzles, laughing with friends, etc.
7 Gratitude: gives God the glory and gives joy to our circumstance.
8 Unless it contributes to your health, do not add. Meaning, take the day at face value. Full of its own demands. Allow that to be enough and do not add anything to the already full schedule.

Let me challenge you to embrace the "I can" as opposed to the "I can't". This can be a hard exercise but one that will give you life and energy. Michael J. Fox says that, "Gratitude makes optimism sustainable." Well, we need to focus on our ability to be grateful. You have survived tough-to-survive circumstances. No one would know because you look so good. So, please embrace the life that you have now. Appreciate the pace. It's OK to miss the former self, to grieve that person. Perfectly alright and necessary. One of our survivor friends said that she does think about her former self but tries not to dwell on it. She would say, "I think about it but don't build a house on it."

A bit about travel and general life experiences. (We will talk more about this in chapter 11, "Events and Holidays".) Traveling will be enough of an energy-drainer, so do your best to take advantage of assistance such as wheelchairs, luggage carts, etc. Also, if you can pre-board, please do. When you choose your seat, please select a place as near the front of the plane as possible. It will eliminate the vibration that comes from sitting in the back of the plane. Also, front seating helps you avoid unnecessary contact with other passengers and luggage.

Here is an escalator and steps hint: have a person you trust stand directly in front of you when going down and directly behind you when going up. This gives you extra trust in case you lose your balance as well as giving you something to look at that doesn't move. Use the handrail located on your stronger side. If your right side is stronger, use the handrail closer to your right side.

The best advice I can give you is to expect the meltdown after a high-intensity event. Too much is being required of you in too short a period. Some of our TBI friends schedule a day of rest after one of those events. You may need more than one day of rest. Some survivors need about three days or more to recover from a stressful event or situation. Do what is best for you. To reduce external stimulus, use a pair of concert earplugs that can block some of the noise/music/sounds. Sometimes, clients use them for church or family gatherings.

Breathing is work. Thinking is work. Please be kind to yourself and give yourself a minute to think about what you want to say. No rushing allowed! Also, you may want to consider keeping your bedroom or another room in the house as a "no clutter" room. It's super-important to not have to navigate through stuff in a place of peace and rest. I understand that the fear of falling is high because of the reality that your balance and sight aren't working at full capacity. Please create as much as possible a clutter-free zone, especially where you spend most of your time. And frankly, if all you have is a chair that is free of clutter, enjoy it! Safe space is needed!

As harsh as brain injury is, please consider being soft with yourself. You will never be lazy. That's not part of your DNA. You have a brain injury. Please rest and listen to your brain and body. Honoring when your brain and body say "stop" will increase your efficiency. Please let love motivate you, not guilt.

In your balcony,
Deana

Homework

- List two deficits and list one coping strategy for each deficit.

_____

_____

- List four things for which you are grateful.

_____

_____

_____

_____

- List one goal that you have since your brain injury.

_____

_____

Resources

Sullivan, C. (2008). *Brain injury survival kit: 365 tips, tools, & tricks to deal with cognitive function loss.* Demos Health.

Zellmer, A. (2015). *Life with a traumatic brain injury: Finding the road back to normal.* CreateSpace Independent Publishing Platform.

3 Family Experience of a Loved One with Brain Injury

Stages of Recovery for Family

The instant a brain injury happens, the family gains a new member: TBI. Of course, one does not realize it at first. During the initial stage, most family members concentrate on getting their loved one all the help needed to heal and recover and get back to functioning at 100%. Unfortunately, whether the TBI is a result from a motor vehicle wreck, an assault, a sports injury, or something else, TBI becomes a permanent part of the family dynamic. Let me share with you some of the stages that a family navigates when TBI is diagnosed. These are stages I've identified in my work with families over the years. Initially, most everyone hopes for full recovery. The perceived meaning of "recovery" is that the person will return to his pre-injury self. It is just a matter of time. I call the first stage: survival. Some of the feelings associated with the first stage are denial and shock. The family is thrust into a new dimension of medical terminology, treatment rehabilitation, and varied expectations. Words and phrases such as "traumatic brain injury", "acute phase of treatment", "deficits", "therapy: physical, speech, occupational", "prognoses", and "aphasia", just to name a few, are thrown around by medical professionals but not given much definition. This first stage is filled with family and friends coming to the aid of their loved ones. It is a time of connection and hope.

After survival, I've noticed that the family experiences disillusionment – the second stage. I believe that families are disillusioned because the progress trajectory of the TBI survivor is not what was initially expected. Being disillusioned is feeling disappointed that the outcome does not match expectations. For example, most people believe that the injured person will bounce back with the right amount of treatment and care. Unfortunately, the recovery pace does not oblige itself to our expectations. At this stage, family members begin to recognize the complexity of brain injury. They may not understand it completely, but they are starting to experience it. For instance, their polite, calm son or daughter exhibits more agitated and less-than-polite behavior. Of course, we know that is because the brain is starting to heal. Yet, because the survivor is not showing their normal personality, it is hard to see that the brain is healing. It is also hard to understand that this is a step of recovery. But as we know, brain injury does not heal like a broken arm heals, with a steady upward route of improvement. It is much more complicated. Disillusionment also means a different understanding of the time of recovery. Especially with brain injury, the healing process can be years long. That is good news and not so good news. It's wonderful that the brain continues to heal. Difficult because it takes time, a long time. Some medical professionals say that the recovery period is two years. However, I have seen the recovery period extend into the 60th year. Neuroplasticity is active and at work. Like reconnecting telephone wires, neuroplasticity reconnects or creates new pathways for the neurons. Sometimes it is hard to see daily change. Improvement is more noticeable in months and years, not days.

After disillusionment, I've noticed that the families start to experience grief. The third stage is called mourning. Once the family member recognizes that their loved one is not going to be the same person, he begins to grieve. This is especially tough when the survivor looks the same as before the injury. TBI is often called an invisible injury because the change is on the inside. So often, survivors do not have an external and obvious sign or scar that shows injury. When the survivor looks essentially the same, it makes accepting brain injury more difficult. Grieving and mourning are complicated because of the traumatic nature of the injury and the mystery of recovery. What does recovery look like? How does someone know that their loved one has reached that recovery point? You may find that the term "recovery" will have different meanings for you and to the survivor. It is not the return of the pre-injury self. However, recovery can mean that the person has surpassed their pre-injury self. I've seen survivors perform at a higher level than they did before their injury. For example, some survivors have become active in legislation and community service on behalf of TBI survivors. I think that the word recovery is best described as the ability to function at one's highest possible level given one's current health and life circumstances. The mourning stage is where you will most likely find yourself angry and/or depressed. That comes with the territory of grief. Anger is a part of this stage and the disillusionment stage too. Bargaining is also common during this stage. It is the act of coming up with scenarios that, if accomplished, would offer a different outcome. For example, asking yourself, "If I had gotten to the hospital faster, would he not have fallen into a coma?" This is a normal reaction to loss.

Another part of the mourning stage is experiencing ambiguous loss. This is the act of grieving what you cannot see. Examples are the passing of milestones of development such as graduations or weddings while in the hospital. The loss of roles in the family is a part of ambiguous grief. Other losses include the loss of routine, purpose, rhythm, and trusting their own brain. One of our mothers said that she kissed her 34-year-old daughter goodbye that morning and kissed her 34-year-old infant in the evening. The motor vehicle crash changed her daughter forever. And it changed the dynamics of their relationship. Partners of TBI survivors grieve the loss of their mate. Not because he is dead but because he is no longer the man she married. Mourning also includes the loss of jobs, friends, expectations. Sometimes, this stage is mourning an actual death, if someone died because of the circumstance such as a motor vehicle wreck or a sports utility vehicle collision. An interesting caveat is that the person dies on a particular date, but the survivor sometimes does not find out until a different date. (Some people in a coma are not aware of the loss.) Many times, the date of discovery is the date of the loss. Our friend, Patti, lost a good friend in the wreck in June. But she did not know it until September. So, September is the date in Patti's mind of her friend's death.

After mourning, I have noticed that the family moves towards adaptation, the fourth stage. This is the stage when the family members actively adjust their behavior and expectations to cope with the deficits of brain injury. This may include coping strategies such as different in-home therapies, managing one's survivor's money, creating social events, participating in vocational rehab, or putting controls on internet access. The understanding of the loved one's brain injury and how it manifests in him is foundational to this step. There may be similarities between brain injury survivors, but each is uniquely different. The adjustments are likely to change as the loved one recovers. For example, impulsiveness can be less manageable at the beginning of the injury, but as the survivor employs his own coping strategies, the impulsiveness may decrease. Another example is when the survivor uses confabulation. This happens in the recovery process and is an attempt by the survivor to make sense of a situation. An example of confabulation is when the survivor remembers A and C but cannot recall B, the middle part, so he makes it up. It is a lie, but it's not meant to deceive but rather to make sense of what happened.

I know that the family has successfully maneuvered through the first four stages when they want to share what they have learned. The fifth and final stage is called service. Once the family learns about brain injury; accepts the reality of it; processes the emotional effects; and creates accommodating strategies, then the family naturally wants to give back or help others. These steps of education, acceptance, processing emotions, and implementing strategies can take months and/or years. Typically, when we as humans overcome or successfully maneuver through a challenging circumstance, we long to share truths learned from the event. To me, this is the restoration part of the experience. Restoring what was lost with a new life of purpose and power is what I've seen with families who have effectively met the challenges of brain injury. We show other people our scars and tell them how we handled the challenges. Several of the TBI friends and their families have become involved in local non-profit organizations about brain injury. Some have become active in legislation to improve medical care or create safety laws. Others have started their own support group. Still others have participated in speaking events for non-profit organizations or churches or community organizations.

Impact on Relationships

The impact of brain injury on relationships can be overwhelming. For parents who have an adult child with TBI, they find themselves reparenting. For spouses of adults with brain injury, they find themselves being more of a parent than a partner. The natural changes in relationships can be extremely challenging. One of the reasons they are challenging is because throughout recovery, the amount of supervision varies depending on the loved one's ability to function. Often, the care partner carries with him/her the image of the injured family member. Many times, the TBI survivors have no knowledge of themselves in the initial stages. Because the memory is traumatic in nature, the care partner is less likely to encourage independence due to fear of another TBI. Transitioning from a caregiver to a care partner is a soft handoff. In other words, it is not an abrupt change. It is working together for the loved one to make safe, independent decisions. Carrie, the wife of a TBI survivor, says that she does not like it when her husband goes on a bike ride. Because he suffered severe TBI from being hit by a car, she is unwilling to accept or be OK with his decision to get back on the bike and ride. It is too risky in Carrie's mind.

As the survivor improves, he can become more of a partner in care. Another example of changing roles comes from Todd. He suffered a TBI from an assault and could not manage his emotions, hold down a job, or interact socially. When his wife was diagnosed with breast cancer, he told himself that he needed to get better to take care of her. What is amazing is that he did improve on all those areas and began being a great support for his wife. He wanted to be the care partner that his wife needed him to be.

Another impact on the relationship involves the maturity aspects. The care partner may notice that the survivor literally grows up as he recovers. Going from an "infant" emotionally to a "teenager" to an "adult" is a long process. Fran, the wife of a brain cancer survivor, said that she has literally watched her husband grow up again. Another example is Richard, the husband of a TBI survivor, who shared that his wife would crawl up into his lap and hug him when she was first injured. He recognized that this was not her normal behavior, but normal for his three-year-old son. Eventually, his wife was able to ask for a hug or affection with adult words and intents. Sometimes the injury adversely affects sexual relationships. Kathy, whose husband suffered two TBIs, said that he was giggly when it came to affection. Another spouse said that she could not have sexual encounters with her husband because he was childlike in his manner. She felt like even though he was an adult, he could not give age-appropriate consent. The flipside of this issue is that some survivors are overly sexualized. This is in part due to the impulsiveness that comes with brain injury. If this is the case, it is best to remove the survivor from the room. Talking to him about appropriate touch or appropriate comments to help circumvent these situations is helpful. Chris experienced a TBI from an assault. After the injury he would tell a woman that he wanted to have sex with her even when he didn't know her. He would also touch a colleague without asking permission, which eventually cost him his job and created legal issues. It is important to communicate that this is inappropriate behavior. Never shame or ridicule the survivor. Simply redirect the behavior. Increased interest in sex or a decreased interest are both common after a brain injury. It is best to seek help with a competent counselor to address these issues. This may be another time to consider working with a competent counselor who understands this aspect of brain injury. In general, counseling helps assist with communication and marital issues. If a counselor is unavailable, consider asking a trusted friend to whom the survivor can be accountable and another friend that the caregiver can be accountable to. By the way, support groups are another outlet to ask for assistance and support.

(Check for groups in your area or online.) And let me suggest that you consider putting your needs and wants back into the equation of caregiving. Too many times, caregivers put themselves last and do not consider what they need. In the beginning, this makes sense. But as time goes on, anger, bitterness, and frustration become as much of a challenge as the brain injury. You are extremely important and deserve to be considered in the situation.

Depression and anxiety plague caregivers in greater numbers than the average population. It makes sense because everything in their lives has changed. From their home life, to work life, to social life...all is different. Often caregivers must quit their jobs or move to part-time status. They are automatically pushed into a role that they have not been prepared for and must know medical jargon that they have never had to know before. Routines have changed. Roles in the relationship are completely different. Friendships are strained due to the inability to keep up with one another as before the injury. Plus, most people do not know what brain injury is or how it affects the family. There is no "normal". Combining that with limited information and limited resources, depression and anxiety are bound to be an issue. The fear of not knowing the future, not understanding the diagnosis, and not recognizing the loved one contributes to anxiety. Experiencing the loss of "normal" and loss of what was and what is to be contributes to depression. Feelings of overwhelm and despondency contribute to both anxiety and depression. The good news is that there is treatment to help with these two mental health issues. Sometimes a physician or psychiatrist may prescribe medication to reduce depression and manage anxiety. Talk therapy such as psychotherapy is very helpful. According to research, both approaches (medication and therapy) practiced in tandem yield the most effective results. However, counseling can be helpful by itself. The key is finding a counselor who understands brain injury and mental illness. Consider interviewing either a psychologist, licensed professional counselor, social worker, or certified brain injury specialist to see if the relationship would be a good fit. I recommend requesting a short consultation for you to briefly share your story and ask how the counselor would help. This will give you a sense of whether the relationship would be a good match for you and your needs. Because the road to recovery of a brain injury is isolating, becoming part of a support group is crucial. Thankfully, there are several support groups online. Depending on one's location and circumstances, finding an in-person support group offers a more intimate connection. Hope After Brain Injury has monthly support groups that meet in person and virtually. On any given month, we will have participants from locations such as England, New Zealand, Canada, California, Florida, Georgia, and Texas.

Often the family needs a connection to the community. Brain injury can absolutely overwhelm the family system, which is why friends, coworkers, and acquaintances are vital to surviving the challenges. As we mentioned earlier, during the initial stages of the injury, community is front and center in that they can provide for immediate and short-term needs of the family. Unfortunately, as time goes on, there is less community involvement. While this makes sense, it still creates isolation. Let this be a call for the community to commit to helping the family long-term. The needs will vary but the ongoing support can make the difference in outcomes. Just as family participation improves the recovery of a survivor, community involvement improves the sustainability of the family. The benefit of community and family collaboration is the increased education and awareness about brain injury recovery. Local religious organizations are a good place to receive assistance. Plus, partnering with a family who is struggling with brain injury can offer insight and understanding that can be applied to other families with similar needs. In the United States, 1 in 300 families are affected by brain injury. So, a church or assembly with average attendance will most likely have more than one family that struggles with brain injury. As a family member, do your best to allow people to help. Do not go it alone. Allow others to help transport your loved one to appointments. Financial needs can be met through gift cards or donations. Emotional and mental needs can be addressed by allowing someone to come sit with your loved one. The caregiver needs a break in the routine to do something for herself. Let's visit with the counselor in her letter to you.

Letter to You

Dear Care Partner,

You are a rock star! Just as survivors are a testament to resilience, you are a testament to devotion. Being faithful even when you don't feel like it is as admirable as recovering from a brain injury. Thank you for loving your survivor well! And remember, you are very important. The research says that the number one factor in successful recovery of a TBI is the presence of family. That is not to put pressure on you but to support your commitment and endeavor to walk alongside your loved one. One of the challenges of loving someone with brain injury is inconsistency. The difficulty you have that he doesn't (sadly) is that you remember the man you married and lived with for so many years.

So, for you, it's a perpetual grieving process. Because of the catastrophic nature of brain injury, you get to pause and reflect about the new you. Dedicate the new relationship to God. Allow Him to shape it. Along with discovery is grief...you may consider writing a letter/journal entry saying goodbye to the former relationship. Put it in a place of honor, not comparison. One of our care partner friends said, "I have been married to two men, and I didn't have to divorce one!" Such a sweet testament of her devotion.

And as you move along this journey, you need cheerleaders not critics. Keep positive people close. Those who do not understand and who tend towards criticism get to do so at a distance. They do not have to be invited into your current walk. Establishing boundaries is protective in nature and always good. "No" is not a four-letter word...it is a great gift to yourself and others. Please use it often and wisely. This will improve your recovery timeline. Saying "yes" when it's not prudent sets us back. You've been set back enough.

Researchers talk about the caregiver burden. Although, as I talk to many in your circumstance, burden is never the word they use. Is it difficult? Absolutely! Is it challenging? A resounding yes! Is it a burden? Not if love is the motivator. So many of you have shared about how complicated brain injury recovery is. The other day I asked a group of caregivers, "What makes you stay?" Each had their own answer of why but all of them said, "Because I love him." Staying is particularly challenging when your survivor does not have empathy or cannot recognize all that you are doing to help. In recovery, though, I've seen that the survivor does develop those skills, if taught. Because the nature of brain injury is self-centeredness, it is difficult to recognize another's participation in and sacrifice for the recovery. However, some survivors see how much their care partner is doing. It depends on where in the brain the injury is and how they are taught to re-engage socially.

The social aspect of recovery is very difficult with most TBI survivors. The cool thing is that when you do find a friend that is willing to understand the injury, you've found gold! Consider the venue and space of a social event. It is difficult to maintain focus when several people are in a small space talking. Cross talk can be confusing and frustrating to someone with TBI. People don't realize that the survivor is burning rubber trying to keep up with the conversation. In the end, it may cost too much to stay. Fatigue will set in...and normally, it hits quickly. Rebuilding relationships is a precious restart. Part of it may include apologies, celebrations, and ponderings for the future. Enter the "new" relationship with openness, understanding, and boundaries. Be OK with stopping inquisitions and entering silence. In other words, allow for silence without asking a bunch of questions. Please consider the same quiet space for yourself as a caregiver. We all need to re-evaluate when we have experienced a huge life change. It's part of the process...painful and lovely all at the same time. The presence of your friends is a huge gift. It's not necessary to fill it with activity. It's OK to laugh, talk, nap, play, and work. The survivor is your priority. You may need to teach others how to comfort you and how to support you. As we mentioned earlier, TBI is a foreign concept to most people. So, they probably need a bit of education to know how to best help and be friends. And one characteristic that I believe is important to discuss is the inconsistency of brain injury. It is consistently inconsistent. That means the progress, the memory, the deficits, the setbacks are all inconsistent. The reason that is important is because most people perceive recovery as an upward trajectory. It is not. When friends say things like, "I understand" or "I have memory problems too," do your best to remember that they are trying to relate, not minimize. It's tough because they really don't get it, and chances are that their memory issue pales in comparison to TBI memory loss. But we can appreciate that they are trying to understand. Remember you are in the middle of a giant reset. So, it will take a minute for you and your friends and family to wrap their minds around how things are different. Your biggest strength is your character, which is made evident by your second-biggest strength, your communication. Trust them both. God will give you the words to say and the wisdom to know when to say them and when to be quiet. Not everyone needs all the details about deficits or particulars about recovery itself. Many of those details are precious to you and your survivor alone. It may be wise to share a statement or two and then let the other person ask questions if they have any. Some questions you may want to answer and some you may not. You get to choose. It's not rude to say, "I wish I could answer that." Or, "That question is for another day."

There is a Hebrew saying: "Let there be such oneness between us that when one cries, the other tastes salt." You are in a silent, sacred space. In that stillness, God meets you. As a survivor, it's a hard place to feel restrained (by limited function ability) and in the oppression of "expectations" (of what you should be able to do). You are free in many ways, yet people (because they are human) expect you to be who you were. It's the drive for homeostasis...balance. When one thing changes, others feel vulnerable. And vulnerability can be met with courage as well as fear. Both are valid. As a care partner of a loved one who has a TBI, you are no longer the same person. That's not good or bad. It just happens when we experience life-changing events.

As you move on this journey, I believe that you will appreciate your strength and abilities more. The other challenge is that your beloved is not aware of his own frailties. In truth, you've been mourning him for quite some time. I think that loving one another through the golden years means extending grace when the other does not have the same capabilities. It's no one's fault. If your love could bring him to wholeness, he would be whole. If his love would bring you to wholeness, you would be whole. Please pray for the Holy Spirit to love your survivor through you (Romans 5:5). Ask for a spirit of calm and peace in your home. Create moments of celebration; moments of reminiscence; and moments of gratitude. And yes, allow yourself the gift of tears.

I want to give you some suggestions when communicating with your loved one, especially early on in the recovery process. It can be difficult to have an extended conversation. When your survivor asks you a question, do your best to answer the questions as briefly as possible. This will take practice. Not giving a lot of explanation is better because more talk requires more processing and can lead to frustration and confusion. The good news is that once you get the hang of it, answering a simple question with a simple answer is more satisfying and productive. Typically, harder conversations are best done in the morning when both parties are fresh and their brains are "online". Please put a timer on the conversation so that it doesn't go long. If possible, keep to one topic only. The challenge is that care partners tend to try to communicate as they did before the injury. It just simply does not work, especially early on. Also, please try to remind yourself not to take your loved one's harshness personally. Try to see it as a symptom of him feeling uncomfortable in some way. Also, responding in his reality will help him feel heard. Using his own words. I guess, it's more of a parrot technique (matching his words) than reflective listening (using different words) but the motivation is love. Please be mindful that your nonverbal matches your verbal. Nonverbal communication accounts for 93% of all communications...so the nouns, verbs, etc. are only 7%! Being mindful of how we are communicating will go a long way towards understanding. So, make sure your tone matches the words. I found that survivors' first language is nonverbal communication. If the survivor responds negatively to what is said, do a quick review to make sure your "audio matches your video" (as Patti Foster says). Another great technique that is hard to master but well worth it if you can: do your best to not take outbursts personally. The reason for not taking it personally is that it is just as likely that something else is bothering your loved one such as sound, lights, etc. Plus, it keeps you from feeling like you need to defend yourself.

This leads to more arguments, typically. You've probably already noticed that trying to reason with someone when he is angry isn't productive. Honestly, the best thing to do is remove yourself from the room or separate yourself in some capacity. Returning to the conversation when your loved one has calmed down will be more productive. During the review of the outburst, you both can come up with a game plan for the next time there is an anger episode. Oh, I thought of something else that could be helpful. Slow down your speed of speech. That normally gives your loved one more time to process what you are saying. Keeping the volume low, energy low, and conversation slower will allow your loved one to stay tuned in to the conversation longer. When talking to your beloved, consider statements like, "Great idea! May we talk about it tonight?" or, "Such a wonderful thought...let's ask a friend to help with that." Or, "Sure. Sounds good." Do your best to preserve your comments.

When there is progress, my recommendation for caregivers like yourself is to helicopter less and drone more. From talking to other caregivers, they communicate that stepping back from watching every move of the survivor can be difficult. It makes sense because of the fear that the survivor will fall or make a mistake that causes him harm. Do your best to adjust the supervision according to the survivor's recovery. So, as you manage the day, give yourself the option to not hover as much as oversee. Of course, this may change throughout the day. But, it's good practice. It's difficult to transition from hands-on care to oversight because you remember what your loved one went through that caused the TBI. Give yourself grace in the process. Before long, you will be able to watch your loved one make safe and healthy decisions. It may take a while, but it will happen.

Here are a few tips provided to you by other care partners. My hope is that you will be able to incorporate a few of them into your routine.

1. Have mercy on yourself. That means to be kind and forgiving. You are doing the best that you can.
2. Ask for help. We talked about asking neighbors or friends to go to the market or run errands for you. It may mean asking someone to stay a couple of hours with your loved one so you can nap.
3. Journal or write. Sometimes people prefer pen and paper, and others prefer making notes on their mobile device. Either way gives you private space for your thoughts. You may find that writing helps you disclose your own thoughts and discover how you are feeling. It is a therapeutic experience.

4. Take your vitamins, eat healthily, and drink water. When you are on "overdrive" emotionally, it releases chemicals in your body that need to be flushed. Drinking water does that. Taking your vitamins and eating healthily give you the needed nutrients to navigate this course. It is another way for you to love yourself and make yourself a priority. Let me add, remember to eat protein to build your system back up from the chronic crises of your loved one's brain injury.
5. Exercise. A better word is movement. If you can incorporate extra steps or movements into your daily routine, I think it will help you reduce your stress and strengthen your body.
6. Schedule a break or time off. Plan to do something for yourself. Whether that is taking a long walk, going window shopping, reading, etc. The goal is to disconnect temporarily from the responsibilities at home.
7. Stay connected to people who understand or want to understand. They can be a lifeline when frustration and agitation enter the equation. Allow them to encourage you. Receive their kindness.
8. Communicate with family, friends, and your survivor. Let the people who have the capacity to listen, listen. They are a rare gift.
9. Seek Godly counsel. If you are unable to share with others your needs and concerns, schedule an appointment with a counselor who is in line with you spiritually and is knowledgeable about caregiving. If the counselor is educated in brain injury recovery, that is a huge benefit.
10. Employ emotional shock absorbers. The following list was created by Tom and Andrea Tatlock, a psychiatrist and his wife, after he sustained a brain injury. The list was added to by Patti Foster, a TBI survivor. The goal is to create a healthy space emotionally. Consider the practice of keeping a:
    a. Sense of gratitude.
    b. Sence of caring and respect.
    c. Sense of reality.
    d. Sense of possibility and hope.
    e. Sense of humor.
    f. Sense of silence.

As I look at these six senses, it reminds me to keep that type of attitude at the forefront. If one's focus is on the problems or deficits, it is extremely hard to see the positives or potential. The sense of reality keeps both of those in focus. It is important to recognize the current challenge of brain injury deficits while keeping the future hope of recovery in mind. Some care partners have said, "I try to see my loved one from a 30,000-foot view and a 3-foot view." And please remember, you are not doing this with your own strength. You have the strength of your Higher Power, those who have gone before you, and your future self.

It is a cool Sunday morning in Arlington, Texas and I am thinking of you. I am praying for God to sustain you and give you courage. I am sending positive thoughts your way, no matter where you are. I want you to know that you are not alone. This journey will certainly make you feel that way, but the Spirit is alive in you. Your connection with your Higher Power will give you strength and direction. The Spirit will empower you to do what is necessary for yourself and for your loved one. Your sacrifice of love is not lost on God. He will honor it. Your devotion is a testament of true mercy. When you don't know what to do, pray. Your faith will guide you.

Until next time,
Deana

Homework

- What do you miss most about your loved one?

_____

_____

- Name four attributes you appreciate about your loved one.

_____

_____

_____

_____

- Name five aspects of you and your caregiving that you appreciate.

_____

_____

_____

- What encouragement would you share with another caregiver?

- Who has inspired you as a caregiver? Explain how.

Resources

Story, L. (2015). *When God doesn't fix it: Lessons you never wanted to learn, truths you can't live without.* Thomas Nelson.

Woodruff, L., & Woodruff, B. (2007). *In an instant: A family's journey of love and healing.* Random House.

Bitsui, R. (2023). *Traumatic brain injury: A caregiver's journey.* Independently Published.

Giffords, G., Kelly, M., & Zaslow, J. (2011). *Gabby: A story of courage and hope.* Scribner.

Carpenter, K., Carpenter, K., & Wilkerson, D. (2012). *The vow: The true events that inspired the movie.* B&H Books.

4 Coping with Anxiety

Anxiety

"I can't trust my own brain." This statement took my breath away when I first heard it. No wonder TBI survivors struggle with anxiety! I cannot imagine what that experience is like. And yet, they work diligently in their recovery hoping that one day they will be able to trust their brain. Depending on the research, almost 40 percent of survivors experience anxiety after a brain injury. Second-guessing decisions is another way anxiety manifests itself. Some of the survivors tend to ask for reassurance when making a decision. It makes perfect sense. If one can't trust his brain, what makes him confident he can make a smart choice or correct choice? Doubting your own brain is not the same as low self-esteem or being insecure. Most people without brain injury misunderstand this behavior as a self-esteem issue.

Anxiety can be a stress reaction. Normally, there are a sense of dread, excessive worry, and irritation. Some people experience poor sleep, muscle tension, or shakiness due to anxiety. Fatigue, restlessness, and poor concentration also accompany anxiety. It is tough to control worry when someone is anxious. To have an official diagnosis of anxiety (generalized anxiety disorder), you must experience these symptoms more days than not for at least six months. Some people describe the symptoms as being nervous or worrying too much.

The care partners also struggle with anxiety more than the general population. Some researchers say that as many as 60 percent of caregivers experience anxiety. This makes sense considering the amount of emotional distress, stress, and chaos that comes with a catastrophic injury. Chronic disability, constant responsibility, feeling overwhelmed or unsure of what to do all contribute to depression and anxiety. While the loved one is trying to recover, all of the responsibilities fall on the care partner. As I've mentioned in chapter 3, I have never heard a care partner consider their loved one a burden. However, dealing with TBI is especially difficult because of the medical jargon, and the multitude of healthcare professionals, therapies, and facilities, all of which must be mastered before returning home. Even though the survivor may recover well, the care partner feels the daily stress and loss of control. Care partners experience a loss of personal time as well as loss of vocational commitment. Some are required to work part-time instead of full-time. Some have to take a leave from work to take care of their loved one. Feeling isolated, unsure, overwhelmed, and ill-equipped contribute to their anxiety. They too experience a loss of independence, loss of self, and loss of prior functioning because their life has completely changed. Financial worries, relationship role changes, uncertainty about the future, and challenges in communication complicate the situation for each care partner.

Loss

Why do brain injury survivors struggle so much with anxiety? Well, other than not trusting your own brain, some of the causes have to do with losses since the injury. The three largest losses are the loss of self, the loss of independence, and the loss of prior functioning. If you think about it, any one of those losses would cause anxiety, much more so all three! We talk more about regaining a sense of self in chapter 12. For now, think with me about what it would be like if, in an instant, you were no longer who you thought you were. That's what it is like for TBI folks. As a TBI survivor, you know this feeling well. I imagine that it is an empty and confusing feeling to lose yourself, to lose who you were in the past. Part of the recovery is learning who you are again. Interestingly, your new self may be different than the pre-injury self. Please embrace the new you.

The loss of independence is a huge adjustment for survivors. One in which many have difficulty, especially when they remember what they could do before the injury. The loss of independence involves physical, psychological, biological, and psychosocial factors. Basically, it means needing assistance in activities of daily living. Most people pride themselves on being able to do things independently. We hesitate to ask for help or accept assistance. Yet, with brain injury, assistance is paramount to recovery. Some examples of loss of independence are: inability to drive, needing assistance taking medication, relying on others to go places and provide necessities for daily living, having a care partner remember appointments on your behalf, and needing assistance to use the restroom or take a bath or make meals. These are a few of the complications of losing independence. As the recovery continues, some of the dependence on others will be reduced. And, with the nature of TBI, there may be an inconsistency in the need for help. For example, if the survivor is feeling less fatigued and more energetic, he may not need help with dressing. These inconsistencies need to be expected and navigated between the survivor and care partner. To do well one day and not the next is simply the pace (and frustration) of TBI recovery.

The loss of prior functioning covers a host of activities from occupation to less structured activities of daily living. In my practice, I hear my clients say, "I used to be able to..." Fill in the blank. Some miss their ability to drive, their ability to make decisions without oversight, to do math, to sign their name without feeling fatigued, to help their partner with the kids, to go to work, or to go grocery shopping without forgetting what to buy. These are just a few examples that show the loss of functioning. One of our survivor friends said that she misses being able to do things spontaneously. Now, she says, she has to think about every step, every decision, and even how to eat. Swallowing is no longer an automatic behavior. Depending on the area of the injury, the survivor may experience losses of function that are different than those experienced by other survivors. As with the other losses, losses of function and independence do tend to improve as recovery continues. The transition of moving towards higher functioning can be challenging for the care partner who tends to want to hover. At times the survivor is ready to make more independent choices and practice functioning at a higher level, but the care partner is slower to "let go of the reins" so the survivor can try on their own. It is a sensitive time for both the survivor and care partner. For example, Simon was injured while riding his bicycle. He had recovered well enough to ride again but his wife was against it. She was remembering the wreck, the severe TBI, the coma of her husband so she did not want him to ride ever again. Yet, for Simon, he wanted to get back on the bike and ride to prove he could and "feel the wind" in his face while he rode. Although reluctant, his wife decided to allow him the experience with precautions in place. She was OK with him riding in the neighborhood but not on a busy street and he was to wear a better helmet. As a couple they were able to navigate his desire for more autonomy. As of this writing, Simon is back competing in local and international triathlons.

Managing Anxiety

Some suggestions on how to manage anxiety. There are several recommendations from different experts in the brain injury and psychology field. One of the most helpful techniques is called mindfulness. This is the practice of being fully present at any given moment instead of concerned about what is going on around us. Staying in the present helps us focus on our breathing and on our body. Concentrating on your breathing is part of mindfulness and anxiety management. Shallower breathing and holding your breath can exacerbate anxiety. If you find yourself sighing, that is a sign that you are not breathing at all or not deeply enough. Sometimes we hold our breath without realizing it. One of the ways you can tell if you are breathing deeply is to watch when you breathe if your stomach rises instead of your chest. A proper deep breath moves your stomach. Inhale through your nose and focus on filling your stomach with air. Exhale through your mouth with pursed lips, visualizing pushing your stomach against your spine. One of the reasons to breathe in through your nose instead of your mouth is that inhaling through your mouth sends a signal to the sympathetic nervous system in your brain that there may be a threat. So, it can contribute to greater anxiety because the brain senses there is a need for a "fight, flight, or freeze" response. Inhaling through your nose activates the parasympathetic nervous system that calms the brain and body. In counseling I teach box or square breathing which originated from pranayama, an ancient breathwork practice from India. The United States Navy SEALs popularized it as they have used it as part of their military stress management program. They refer to it as tactical breathing technique, used to help the soldiers deal with high-stress situations in battle and combat. Here are the steps for box breathing:

1. Inhale through your nose while mentally counting to four.
2. Hold your breath to the count of four.
3. Exhale through your mouth while mentally counting to four.
4. Hold your breath to the count of four.
5. Repeat steps 1–4 four times.

For some folks four seconds is too long; if so, try to practice box breathing while counting to two seconds or three seconds at each step. Ideally, the exercise takes about one to one and a half minutes. I suggest to my clients to practice throughout the day so that when they feel anxious, the technique can become second nature.

Education on brain injury and what a typical recovery trajectory may look like helps care partners manage their anxiety. Fran, whose brother had a TBI, said that she wanted two things primarily: education and resources. Having a better understanding of what brain injury is and what to expect in recovery can circumvent some of the anxiety associated with caregiving. Let me share an experience that happened to two of our care partners. Susan was told that her daughter would have to be transferred to acute rehabilitation to continue her treatment. Her daughter was coming out of a coma. The physician warned Susan that her daughter, a religious young lady, may use words (profanity) she did not use before the injury. So, when her daughter gained consciousness, she did curse "like a sailor" which is part of the injury, not her character. Susan appreciated the warning of what to expect and was not nearly as concerned as she could have been without the information. Robert was told that his wife would be discharged from an acute hospital for rehabilitation. He had to research where to take his wife. The transfer facility was of little help. As his wife became more aware of her surroundings, she was easily irritated and confused. She yelled at him and the staff. He became upset, took her accusations personally, and couldn't spend time with her without getting angry himself. Because no one told him that when the brain is injured, his wife will experience more anger and frustration and will probably take it out on whoever is with her, he took her statements personally and reacted in anger. He struggled with additional anxiety because of not understanding what was happening with his wife.

Support groups and connections with family and friends can soften the caregiving responsibilities and help alleviate the loneliness. Search the internet for support groups that can be attended online or in person. As of this writing, there are several support groups available on social media. Once connected with a support group, treat it as a family. They will be a lifeline of support as you traverse the recovery journey. Listening to podcasts and reading are two more resources of education and support. A list of books is located in the Additional Resources.

If you have flown in an airplane, you hear the directions of putting on your own oxygen mask before helping someone else. This is a great example of self-care. Managing anxiety incorporates making one's own health a priority. Exercise, taking medication, journaling, adequate sleep, healthy eating, and relaxation are all important. Walking in nature particularly is helpful for anxiety because of several factors. One is that being in the sun helps increase energy. Experiencing nature, whether it is listening to the wind or birds or watching ducks in a pond, can offer a different perspective. It reminds the care partner that he is not alone, and that life is bigger than the current circumstances. Sometimes nature helps people connect to their Higher Power. Lastly, accessing help is essential to long-term health in the care partner journey. Some prefer to shoulder all of the responsibilities alone but, unfortunately, this will shorten one's effectiveness. "Ask help and receive help" is a recommendation one of our survivors passed along to the care partners.

Positive outlook, relaxation techniques such as imagery and meditation, and reframing our thoughts are three other ways to manage anxiety. A positive outlook is a mindset. Hope is the fuel. Dr. Andrew Maas, a neurosurgeon from Belgium who was awarded the Lifetime Achievement Award in 2016 by the International Brain Injury Association, said in a private interview that hope "is as essential as breath". I believe he is right. How can a healthcare professional work effectively without keeping hope in the recovery picture? In my professional opinion, it is malpractice to say a TBI survivor has no recovery after two years. This is untrue. As I have had the honor of working with and knowing survivors of all ages, they continue to improve and make strides towards recovery for years and years after the initial injury. It is vital that we as part of the brain injury community demonstrate a positive, encouraging, hope-filled manner as part of our value system. Hope is medicine. Please understand, I am not advocating blind enthusiasm but rather foundational belief that while we are alive our body and brain are working to improve. Sometimes our families come to us with little or no hope that things will get better. Borrow mine. I have all the hope in the world that your circumstances will change and change for the better. And then I have the privilege of walking with them on their journey for as long as they will have me.

Imagery or relaxation techniques are helpful in managing anxiety. Patti Foster, a TBI survivor, voiced a wonderful guided imagery exercise written by me. It is called "Visualization – Cloud" and the script has been provided to you (see appendix A). There are many other imagery exercises easily accessible through an internet search. Relaxation exercises help relax the body and quiet one's thoughts. They help to reduce blood pressure and decrease stress and muscle tension. One of the techniques is progressive muscle relaxation. This exercise takes the listener through a series of noticing different muscle groups, tightening them, and then releasing the tension in a methodical, easy manner. Again, there are several types of relaxation exercises available on the internet. The art of meditation is practiced in several worldwide religions as a part of their preparation to worship. It helps to focus your thoughts and concentrate on your breathing while visualizing a Divine Presence. Christianity uses meditation as a form of prayer reflecting on passages in the Bible. Judaism practices meditation in directing one's heart to G-d. Hinduism uses yoga to prepare the body for meditation and prayer. Meditation is utilized in Buddhism as a practice of paying attention to the body, breathing, and thoughts.

A technique of cognitive-behavioral therapy is called cognitive restructuring. Simply put, it is the practice of reframing a thought. It helps people change the way they think about a situation or a belief. Look at your room. Is there a picture hanging on the wall? Think about changing the frame around the picture. Would that also change how you feel and believe about the picture? Chances are it would make a difference. That's an analogy of what reframing means. A couple of examples to consider. If you have a friend who tends to dig in their heels and be headstrong, we could say that the person is stubborn, which would have a negative connotation or meaning. Or we could describe the person as tenacious, which offers a more positive description. Another example is when one of your friends is late for a lunch meeting. You could think that the friend is being lazy, unorganized, or disrespectful to not attend the appointment. How would you feel about your friend if that is the belief of why he is late? Probably very negatively. However, let's say your friend comes to lunch late and apologizes because he was caught up in an emergency with his neighbor. Through this reframing (your belief of what happened), you are kinder and more receptive to your friend instead of offended. One of my colleagues said that reframing is one of his most effective coping strategies. I have also found it helpful when working with people. It automatically changes a potentially anxious situation to one where we can practice grace. Our friend Rosa, Holocaust and TBI survivor, was exceptional at reframing (although I am not sure she identified it formally). In a private conversation I asked her, how did she survive the war? She responded by saying, "I wanted to see who won? And, you know what? I won. Hitler is dead. Israel became a state. And I have two sons and three grandchildren." Although she lost all of her family in Auschwitz and was severely beaten by Josef Mengele, she chose the perspective of seeing things in light of her benefit. One last example that may hit closer to home. Let's say your TBI survivor kept forgetting what you have told him multiple times. One way of interpreting the memory issues is to think he didn't care, or he would remember. Or you could remind yourself that he has brain injury, which means he has trouble with short-term memory loss. Forgetting is not a character or behavior issue, it is an injury issue; therefore, help the survivor with written notes or by keeping a whiteboard in easy view to help him remember.

Let's see what else may be helpful in managing anxiety. May I invite you to the counseling room?

Letter to You

Dear Friend,

Anxiety or chronic nervousness or excessive worry are hard! It comes with recovering from brain injury because of all the changes now a part of your life. Just know that you are not doing anything wrong, this is just part of the process for some survivors. We can think about ways to manage the anxiety or at least reduce some of its power. For example, instead of saying, "I am anxious," try saying, "Part of me is anxious." This helps reduce its power. Plus, it helps you not feel powerless over it. Another technique is acknowledging that you are feeling anxious but being curious about it. Implicit memory is the feelings or body memories. When there is fear or anxiety, be curious about it. What is the anxiety trying to say? Curiosity eliminates the judgement. Remember that sometimes anxiety appears when we are overwhelmed. So, maybe the anxiety is saying you may be doing too much. Figuring out the trigger is half the battle. It is common for people to say they feel anxious but cannot figure out what triggered it. So, think about when you started feeling anxious and what happened at the time. Think about why you are feeling anxious and why now? You may consider not reading or listening to anxiety-producing information. And reminding yourself of what is true this minute. Meaning, right now I am safe. I have plenty to eat. I have a loving wife/husband. I have a nice home. The "what-ifs" exacerbate anxiety. So, replace the "what if" with "what is".

Lack of quiet can cause anxiety. I know that life happens around us. Sometimes when we can't get away, we can distract our senses. For example, having a program on the radio/TV that is Zen for you. Research says that the sound of loons helps relax and settle anxiety in people. Maybe there is a sound that you particularly enjoy. As you practice quiet and deep breathing, consider repeating a phrase to help you stay grounded. For some, a Bible verse is helpful. Others use a confirmation such as, "I am safe and protected." "I have everything I need." You may create your own message that settles you.

Basically, anxiety is fear. Fear is a perfectly normal feeling considering your circumstances and challenges. Concentrating on the fear tends to make it larger instead of smaller. So, it is more effective to focus on what is true and what you can control. One of our survivors was unable to drive after her injury. She could not walk outside without losing her balance. When she became anxious, she mapped out a path in her house to walk. She would "furniture surf" when walking to keep her balanced. To her, this small bit of control helped her feel less anxious.

Just a few reminders on how to manage anxiety:

1. If it's too hot to enjoy outside, imagine it. Imagine the wind, a cool breeze, a waterfall. Creating the oasis in your head has as much benefit as actually being in the environment.
2. Deep breathing. I've noticed that sometimes you breathe shallowly and/or hold your breath. Try to be mindful of deep breaths. Practice square or box breathing described earlier in the chapter.
3. Distraction. Thinking or doing something else can break the anxiety cycle.
4. Grounding. Tune in to the visuals, sounds, and textures of your surroundings.
5. Reduce the external stimuli as much as possible. When one feels anxious, noise/lights/talking makes it worse.
6. Exercise with caution.
7. Focal point. Sometimes having something to focus on relieves your mind and settles your emotions.
8. Rest when you can't sleep. Do your best to not require yourself to do and go.

If you think about it, recovering from brain injury makes you a bit of an expert on a lot of therapies! Managing anxiety is no exception. Make sure you are eating healthily and getting enough sleep. If you need a rest, do it! I don't mean to be insensitive here but laugh when you can. I know that brain injury is no laughing matter but sometimes humor is the small bubbles of joy we need to manage anxiety.

Just breathe,
Deana

Homework

- Make a list of what triggers your anxiety.

_____

_____

_____

_____

- Make a list of things you can do that will help reduce anxiety.

_____

_____

_____

_____

Resources

Vaishnavi, S., & Rao, V. (2023). *Healing the traumatized brain: Coping after concussion and other brain injuries.* Johns Hopkins University Press.

Coetzer, R. (2018). *Anxiety and mood disorders following traumatic brain injury: Clinical assessment and psychotherapy.* Routledge.

5 Coping with Depression

Depression

Depression is one of the most common mental health issues in the United States. In fact, research says that as many as 18 percent of adults experience some kind of depression in their life. Symptoms such as low mood, poor energy, problems with sleep, difficulty concentrating, and diminished self-worth that are present for two weeks or more can signify depression. Of course, one will want to seek professional help when and if these symptoms are present or worsen. Calling emergency services, going to the local emergency department, or contacting your healthcare provider are all important interventions especially if one is feeling suicidal, hopeless, or despondent.

Depression can be debilitating although not always. Very influential people through the years have experienced depression yet been able to accomplish huge feats. For example, Abraham Lincoln suffered from depression (melancholia, as it was known then) and was able to lead the United States during the Civil War. Winston Churchill led the world in its defeat of Hitler during World War II while dealing with what he referred to as "the black dog" of depression. Isaac Newton, Vincent van Gogh, and Ludwig van Beethoven all experienced daily depression. More recent personalities who reported significant depression are Michael Phelps (the most decorated Olympian in US history), J.K. Rowling (author of the Harry Potter series), and Dolly Parton (queen of country music). Phelps admitted himself into a mental health inpatient facility to help him deal with his depression. Rowling wrote of her experience with depression in the form of Dementors in her book. Parton turned to her faith in God to help her through the depression. With proper care, one can function highly even with the presence of depression.

Caregivers go through depression too. Research says that the rate of depression in caregivers of TBI survivors can be twice as high as in the normal population. Whether a spouse, parent, child, or sibling, they feel the responsibility of taking care of their loved one with brain injury and yet do not have the knowledge of what to do or who to ask. Caregivers need resources and practical tips on how to manage brain injury. It is a journey no one wants to take yet here they are. Too often they feel the loss of family and friend support. There is marital strife and dissatisfaction due to the stress and burden of caregiving. They do their best to manage the emotional and behavioral challenges of their brain injury survivor but often feel depleted and discouraged. It feels as though their best effort is not enough. The feeling of inadequacy contributes to depression. Because of the severity and chronicity of the injury, caregivers experience financial strain, role changes, expectation adjustments, as well as a host of adverse effects to the family system. Lack of empathic communication, misunderstanding, and lack of patience compound the emotional toll it takes on the caregiver. The relationship with the survivor changes indefinitely. A support group or counselor who understands the complexities of brain injury will help mitigate some of the depression associated with caregiving. Chapter 3 dives into more detail of the experience of a family member when brain injury enters the picture. Offering problem-solving education specific to brain injury, emotional support, and counseling are key intervention strategies for caregivers. Fran, sister of a TBI brother, said that what she wanted when he was first injured were "education and resources". So often, family members are not given the information they need to properly care for their loved one. This lack of assistance contributes to depression and helplessness.

So, what does depression look like? Although it is different for every person, there are commonalities. Having no energy and feeling fatigued and tired can be a hallmark of depression. The kind of tiredness that sleep does not remedy. Sometimes people with depression sleep multiple hours a day and sometimes they only sleep two to three hours per night. Either way, there is poor rebound and limited to no energy. Tearfulness can be a part of depression as well as feeling too bad to cry. It is as though there is no feeling whatsoever. Some say that they feel completely numb. Others say that they feel like a robot just going through the motions. Depression takes away the desire to do things or to enjoy activities. No energy coincides with no appetite. Again, the opposite can be true as well. Some eat incessantly. Others cannot eat at all. Pervasive sadness is another characteristic of depression. The difference between depressed sadness and grief-related sadness is that in grief, one knows the reason (a death) for the sadness. In depression, there is no one thing that causes the feeling. It is everything and nothing, if that makes sense. Also, helplessness and hopelessness go hand in hand with depression. Questions like, "What's the use?" or, "Will I ever feel good again?" are common. It is important for loved ones to pay attention to the statements and questions of someone depressed. One may reach out to professionals on their loved one's behalf, especially if there is a worry of self-harm. Again, if the depression lasts more than two weeks, professional help is warranted.

Managing Depression

Treatment for depression can range from inpatient hospitalization to outpatient counseling. Weekly group therapy has proven effective in developing coping strategies and eliminating the isolation that often accompanies depression. Sometimes medication is given to help alleviate or lessen the symptoms of depression. There are certain counseling techniques that have proven effective in working with this issue. Cognitive-behavioral therapy (CBT) is considered the gold standard of treatment. Briefly, CBT helps the individual recognize how their thinking affects how they are feeling and how they are doing, which contributes to a depressive episode. The therapist or counselor will help identify cognitive distortions such as black-and-white/all-or-nothing thinking, catastrophizing (imagining situations are worse than they are), or other ways of thinking that feed depression or make it worse. Once those distortions are identified, the counselor can help the individual change their way of thinking to a more truthful and realistic perspective. For example, a client may say that he is depressed because, "Nothing ever works out for me." This is a type of overgeneralization whereby one makes broad assumptions from a few events. Fortune telling is when one believes without sufficient evidence that a situation will turn out badly. An example would be, "I'm not applying for that job because I know they won't hire me." Mind reading is another common cognitive distortion. This happens when one assumes he knows what someone is thinking or feeling. For example, "I don't like eating in a restaurant alone because everyone thinks I'm a loser." These are a few examples of how our thinking about situations can negatively affect how we feel and, therefore, how we behave. When one manages his/her thoughts, the feelings associated with the thought will adapt to the more useful idea. At that point, the person makes healthier decisions that help improve their situation. Cognitive distortions I see in brain injury are statements like, "It's been two years since my injury and I'm not going to get any better." Of course, this is not true. We have seen improvement in brain injury survivors up to decades after the initial injury. Recovery just seems a bit slower than during the first few months. An alternative to the negative statement is, "I am improving slowly whether I see it or not."

Another form of treatment is psychotherapy. In psychotherapy the individual works with a psychotherapist weekly to share feelings and past experiences. It is commonly referred to as "talk therapy". The therapist will offer insights into possible causes of behavior. The client and therapist work together to create coping strategies and possible solutions to the stated problem. Opportunity is given to gain insight into behavior and practice more healthy decisions. Typically, it is a long-term process whereby one meets with the therapist weekly for an extended period. Research shows that talk therapy and medication are the most effective ways of dealing with depression.

Depression and Brain Injury

What about depression and brain injury? Are they related? Depression with brain injury can be both physical and emotional. The organic changes in the brain structure coupled with the emotional losses and changes both contribute to a distinct type of depression. Unfortunately, the depression rate in survivors of brain injury is higher than in the normal population. Depending on the research, it is said to affect as many as 50 percent of brain injury folks. Sadly, depression can be just as prevalent seven years post-injury due to the extended period of lower-than-expected function. Depression may come and go in the recovery process. Some symptoms one may experience (along with those previously mentioned) are not wanting to be around others, feeling worthless, moving or speaking more slowly, or feeling like a failure. Distinct to some brain injury is the frustration due to the difficulty of learning, or not being motivated by pleasurable activities. This is seen through impulsiveness and easily becoming frustrated. Again, if these symptoms last longer than a couple of weeks, it is wise to consider professional help. Connect with one's primary physician, a neurologist, or physiatrist for assistance or referrals to psychiatric/mental health professionals that know brain injury. Because the brain circuitry is different from an injury, it is important for the healthcare provider to be experienced in working with brain injury as well as depression so that the medication (if needed) is monitored appropriately.

Some of the reasons for the prevalence of depression are due to the immense changes that occur with brain injury along with the structural changes of the brain itself. For example, some experience depression because of the location of the injury in the part of the brain that controls emotion. Early in brain injury, one may experience mood swings or bouts of crying or laughing. Those are different from a depressive episode. Typically, those behaviors are temporary and will settle down to more appropriate expression as the brain heals. Sometimes there is a change in the natural chemicals in the brain. Some of the emotional reasons for depression specific to brain injury are the adjustment forced by a temporary or lasting disability, dealing with a possible loss of roles in the family and work and in society, or not knowing how to fit into the world. Facing an unknown future can be daunting for survivors. Lastly, if there is a genetic disposition towards depression in the family or a history of abuse, there is a higher likelihood that the survivor will experience it. Also, substance abuse or financial and legal issues may arise after brain injury. These socioeconomic factors may contribute to a depressive episode. To consider these other aspects of depression, let's talk about depression from the counselor's perspective.

Letter to You

Dear Friend,

Even though I hate that you are going through this, I know that depression is part of the healing process. One thing to remember is that having depression does not mean you are crazy. It can mean that you are probably beyond your normal resources to manage stress, or you are overwhelmed with all the changes in your life. It sort of comes with the territory of brain injury. You have a right to be depressed. It makes complete sense. When one's life is turned upside down or comes to a complete halt, depression is bound to be a result. It may help you to remember that some of the greats in history experienced it too. Remember King David in the Psalms? During one of his depressive episodes, he asked God to put his tears in God's tear bottle (Psalm 56:8). He is asking God to hold dear his pain and agony. God holds you close too. Remember that verse Psalm 34:18? God says that He will hold the brokenhearted close to Him. That's you. The psalter in Psalm 88:18 (New International Version) says that, "darkness is my closest friend." That's depression! Even Jesus experienced despair in the Garden of Gethsemane (Matthew 26:36–

46). You probably know someone among your family and friends who knows what depression feels like. You are not alone. Please know that it will get better. And if you ever get to a place where you are thinking about suicide or wanting to hurt yourself, please tell a family member or call emergency services. They will help you.

Sometimes depression is a phase of the healing process. At this stage of your recovery, you want to see depression as a good thing. Not that it feels good but that it is a necessary part of healing. This type of depression comes from realizing the difference between what you used to do and what you can do now…that is a huge difference. Having the awareness that there are distinct differences is why this is considered progress. Try to see it as a part of the grieving process. It will improve as you recover. It helps to remember that this will pass. See it as a step in the recovery journey. You may consider writing about your feelings about the various losses you have experienced. It is good to write. The act of putting something on paper helps sort out your feelings. And it helps to say what you are thinking without interruption from someone else. Plus, it helps to have a journal entry that you can go back to and reference.

When depression is part of the grieving process, it is important to give yourself the space to process the loss. Ambiguous grief is the loss of something you cannot touch like the loss of function, vision, dreams, roles in life, your former self. (You may want to read or reread Chapter 8 on "Grief and Ambiguous Loss".) It is also the loss one feels when someone is physically there but psychologically absent. For example, you look the same, but you are not the same. As we mentioned, the loss of function is huge. Not being able to do the things that you used to do or want to do. For example, it is hard when you need someone to oversee your daily activities just to make sure you are safe. I do think that as you recover, the need for moderate supervision will diminish. You will become more independent. Please be patient with yourself. Where you are is not where you will stay. Neuroplasticity (reconnecting and/or finding new pathways between axons and dendrites within the brain) is working on your behalf.

With the loss of function comes the loss of the various roles we have in our lives. Things that you used to do before the injury are either not possible or too difficult. Something as small as taking out the trash or doing the laundry can be a challenge. These are times when depression can hit especially hard. Not being able to return to work is another loss and role change. One of our TBI friends explains it this way: "I've moved from being the father and provider to another kid my wife has to take care of." That's tough! Thankfully, he sees that his change in roles is helpful in different ways. For example, he can take the kids to school, which he couldn't do before. It does help to know that although roles and functions change, it does not mean you cannot contribute. Please remember that some losses can be temporary. Processing these changes and losses can take their toll. Sometimes there is a loss of vision or dreams. Perhaps you had dreams of retiring early and traveling with your partner and now those dreams are gone. Grieve those. Just because they didn't happen doesn't mean they weren't important and a part of you. And in your grief, please consider creating new dreams and new goals. Grief opens the door to restoration and creativity. Cry the tears of loss but don't stop short of dreaming new dreams. Above all, please be gracious to yourself.

You may notice that depression comes after an angry episode. This too is normal for a TBI survivor. One of our TBI friends says that after he has an outburst, he becomes "down and in a dark place because that did not used to be me. I could handle my anger better." Some survivors feel low and sad from the instant they wake up from the coma or have a recognition that something has changed. One of our friends said that she has experienced depression since waking from her coma. Her family told her that she would often ask, "Where's my happy?" In her experience depression is always present, but not always at the same degree. She said that it tends to show itself with fatigue and exhaustion. You may monitor the episodes for yourself to see if you can identify a trigger or pattern. Because every brain injury is unique, one's depression may also be unique in the way it shows itself. So, please put on your investigative hat and see if you can recognize trends of your experience with depression. I think that will help you feel more in control of it and give you direction on what changes may be necessary to alleviate it or reduce its impact. You may recognize that depression comes in stages before a recovery spurt of improvement.

So, what do you do when you feel depressed? Acknowledge it. That may sound strange but acknowledging it will lessen its power. Be curious about it. Ask yourself, "Why is depression present now?" See if you can work out what it is trying to say. For example, maybe it is telling you to slow down. Depression tends to isolate so do your best to be around someone you trust. Someone's presence is sometimes all you need. Go for a walk. If you can navigate safely, exercise is helpful. Not the workout kind of exercise. I'm talking about simple movements. One of our TBI friends would walk around a path in the house. She called it "furniture surfing" because she had to hold on to a piece of furniture to keep her balance. But it helped her move. It gave her a goal and made her feel productive. Another strategy is to go outside. Being in the sunshine for at least ten minutes per day will help your brain. The researchers say that regular exposure to the sun improves one's immune system, helps the brain boost serotonin (a neurotransmitter that improves mood) production, supports bone health, lowers blood pressure, and provides various other health benefits. Rosa, our friend who suffered a TBI as a Holocaust survivor, would sit outside for 20 minutes a day. She said that it helped her feel better and less sad and discouraged. Also, being outside, enjoying nature helps change one's perspective. Sometimes depression gives us tunnel vision. Feeling the wind and listening to the birds reminds us that there is a bigger world and expands our vision. (That reminds me, listening to loons has been said to help alleviate anxiety too!) If it is a rainy, overcast day, light therapy lamps can do the trick. Finally, talking to someone who understands can be very effective in not feeling alone. So, companionship, exercise, and the sun are three natural ways that will lessen depression. Give it a go. I'm cheering you on!

Walking with you,
Deana

Homework

- Chart episodes of depression. See if you can identify any trends.

  _____

  _____

- Journal. Writing down your thoughts serves two purposes: expression and discovery. Many times, the act of writing will reveal other aspects of depression or the situation that will offer insight into how to manage it.

  _____

  _____

- Make a list of your goals. It's OK if they are small. Try to come up with at least four.

  _____

  _____

  _____

  _____

Resources

Foster, P. (2016). *Hope for the journey: A 52-week spiritual journal.* Redemption Press.

Arthur, M. (2022). *Embracing hope after traumatic brain injury: Finding Eden.* Routledge.

6 Coping with Anger

Anger and Brain Injury

When someone experiences a brain injury, their emotional expression is adversely affected. The reason is that the emotional center of the brain has been damaged. One may notice that there is a general inability to manage emotions after traumatic brain injury (TBI). Anger is mostly directed at family and friends. Not because they deserve it but because they are the safest outlets for it. Expressing anger in social or employment situations could lead to rejection or worse. So, it is best for the family and friends to understand the reason and not take it personally. One of the most common emotional responses after brain injury is anger. Research notes that up to 75 percent of TBI survivors struggle with anger or have a short fuse. Sometimes it is a stage in recovery and sometimes it is a permanent result that the survivor must learn to navigate through behavior modification or medication management. As opposed to happiness or sadness, anger can lead to destructive or inappropriate behaviors such as yelling, cursing, throwing things, or physical acting out. Todd was injured as a stuntman at a popular amusement park. After his injury, he struggled to manage his anger. One day his anger went unchecked and as he was driving, he became angry at his wife and intentionally flipped the vehicle. Later, he admitted that he was trying to harm her. Todd started working with a psychiatrist who specialized in brain injury. With medication and psychotherapy he was able to avoid such outbursts.

The areas of the brain that predominantly manage emotions are the frontal lobe and the limbic system. The frontal lobe controls executive functions such as problem-solving and impulse control. The limbic system, made up of the amygdala, hypothalamus, hippocampus, and limbic cortex, manages emotional control and processes. (For more details about the limbic system, read chapter 1, "What is Brain Injury?") The limbic system also helps one make sense of the world. During the acute phase of recovery (first few weeks), anger might be difficult, if not impossible, to control. It is important for the survivor to remember it is the brain injury, not that he is a bad person. Confusion can lead to anger outbursts. One physician warned the family that their daughter, a dedicated Christian young lady, may say things that they might never have heard her say. And, indeed, the cursing coming from this woman came as a shock. However, they knew that this wasn't their daughter, it was the brain injury. Other family members have shared that their loved one acted completely out of character after the brain injury. Especially in the early stages, one may experience their loved one becoming belligerent, forceful in their opinion, or behaving irrationally. The wife of a doctor who had a brain injury said that her husband would try to escape the rehabilitation facility because he did not think he belonged there. The anger and its behavior are because the brain is damaged and trying to heal. Especially if there is damage in the orbitofrontal lobe (behind the forehead and by the eye) and certain areas of the brain that manage emotions, anger can be hard to control or manage. As survivors recover, they can learn and practice coping skills to manage it.

Anger can also be a healthy step towards recovery. It just feels miserable. There are three levels of anger: anger turned inward (also considered depression), general anger at the world (better but not great expression), and anger directed towards the person/situation that created the emotion (most healthy expression). In recovery, notice which level of anger the survivor is exhibiting. This will give insight into why the anger is expressed the way it is. Thinking of it as a map can help take some of the sting out of it and give direction. In other words, think of anger as a point in the day. What is it saying? Where did it come from? Where will it take you? Please consider using anger to give yourself a voice. The energy in anger can be used productively, to help you meet a need or discuss a concern. Do your best to not use the energy to hurt yourself or someone else.

Triggers of Anger

Anger can also be triggered by physical or emotional discomfort. Physical disabilities or challenges tend to frustrate the person. Learning to walk again or feed themselves or any other function of daily living takes quiet and patience. When the survivor feels pressured or simply frustrated that his own body is not cooperating, an anger outburst is likely. Pain also tends to exacerbate angry episodes. A severe TBI survivor said that he must live from pain pill to pain pill. He said that the pain kept him from wanting to talk or engage in therapy. Fatigue and overstimulation contribute to a short fuse. A rule to remember with brain injury is that fatigue exacerbates most anger responses. If one can manage one's fatigue, one can more easily manage the anger. (Check out chapter 10, "Fatigue and Rest", for more details.) This may mean scheduling naps during the day or retreating to a quiet space.

Overstimulation is another possible trigger of angry outbursts. This means that the survivor has too much external stimulus. For example, being in a crowded room or listening to multiple conversations can be overstimulating. Often room temperature, sounds, and lighting can trigger an outburst. Room lighting may be too bright. Consider lower-wattage lamps instead. This trigger is the easiest to remedy. It is best to lower the lights, turn down or turn off the television, stereo, or electrical devices. Ask the family and friends in the room to speak slowly and one at a time. When there is too much to process at any one moment, frustration occurs. It may be helpful to have a designated quiet area for your loved one. Lower stimuli help the survivor settle down and regroup. One of the TBI survivors would become fatigued and overwhelmed during a dinner with friends. He would excuse himself and rest for a few minutes and then rejoin them. Part of overstimulation is asking the brain injury survivor to do more than one thing at a time. For example, it is unwise to carry on a conversation when he is trying to walk. Let the main thing be the main thing. This means that the caregiver needs to slow down and be mindful of what the survivor is trying to do.

Perceived insults may trigger an angry event. This can be from the concrete thinking and literal thinking of a brain injury survivor. He may not understand an abstract statement and perceive it literally. Irritability may also be the result of slowed cognitive processing. In conversation, the survivor may not be able to process the dialogue as quickly as his counterpart. Also, he may interrupt because he does not want to forget his thoughts. So, it is very helpful for the person speaking with a TBI survivor to speak slowly, remembering the processor is a bit slower. Additionally, recognizing the role of nonverbal communication can go a long way in alleviating some of the misinterpretations. One survivor stated that nonverbal communication was her first language after the injury. She read the body language, facial expressions, tone, and gestures before processing the words. As a former media personality, she shared the importance of "letting your audio match your video".

Managing Anger

Dealing with anger in someone who has suffered a TBI can be very challenging. It can often feel like the caregiver is walking on eggshells waiting for the next outburst. The best way to manage anger is to understand what causes it. Triggers of anger can be related to lack of independence and autonomy. For example, if the survivor depends on someone else for their care or if the survivor cannot make decisions by himself without the input from family. Not being released to drive is particularly difficult for survivors who remember they drove prior to their brain injury. Regaining that function may require driving classes. It is helpful to remember that the survivor is getting better and learning to manage his anger.

Not being able to participate in valued activities can be frustrating. One survivor stated that he really dislikes it when someone tells him what to do. He said, "I'm just getting my brain back. Let me use it." The desire to use one's own brain is an important point for caregivers to remember. Almost universally, survivors (as well as non-injured people) do not like it when someone tells them what to do. As a survivor friend said, "I'm learning to live again. Don't do my thinking for me." Walking the fine line of allowing the survivor autonomy while keeping him safe can be difficult. It's important to celebrate the small victories of independence. This keeps the recovery steps in mind and communicates hope of future improvement. An example of future improvement would be something as simple as doing their own grooming or making their own cereal. As a caregiver, do not try to interpret anger with a specific intention or motive because, typically, there is no intent behind the anger. Another thought, try not to be too helpful. This is another fine line because helping may be perceived as control.

For the caregiver, managing anger means not taking aggressive behavior personally. If the loved one becomes defensive, arguments will surely ensue. The TBI survivors cannot process objectively when angry nor can they reason when they are angry. Most people have trouble processing information when in an elevated emotional state. Interestingly, when someone is angry, he is accessing a different part of the brain. That is why the survivor may be slow to speak in a calmer state but very quick, deliberate, and focused when angry. Survivors may or may not have trouble with problem-solving, memory, slowed thinking, and poor focusing, which all contribute to the difficulty in understanding their behavior. Taking the statements and behavior personally is not always accurate. Sometimes it is helpful to think that the brain is angry. Even though the survivor is yelling at you doesn't mean they are angry with you. It is more effective to approach the outburst with an investigative posture. What triggered the event? What can be done to avoid arguments in the future? It is best to not argue or engage with the survivor who is angry. Typically, the interaction escalates anger and behavior. It is best to withdraw. As I often say, take the energy out of the room. This takes the pressure off both parties and helps each other calm down. After the episode, consider creating a strategy about what to do should the situation happen again. Open communication and dialogue without judgement go a long way towards understanding the outburst and hopefully mitigating it in the future. Sometimes comments are received better than questions. Some survivors feel pushed into a corner with questions because their brain is working hard to keep up with the conversation. Statements like, "That was tough, huh?" or, "Thanks for telling me" can open the door for more communication. Oh, and do your best to not step on silence. Most people are not comfortable when someone hesitates to say something or there is a perceived time lapse. Giving the survivor space and time to think goes a long way in helping them feel heard and understood. For more insights into anger and brain injury, let's listen to the counselor.

Letter to You

Dear Friend,

One of the challenges of TBI is the short fuse of irritability and anger. I know that you have dealt with that in the past and still struggle at times now. Please know that this is partially because your brain is healing. Typically, anger comes out in sharp comebacks or long diatribes or rants. Giving yourself a minute to breathe, pause, or walk away helps with this. Try to notice changes in your body when you are getting angry. One of the signs that anger may be building is an increased heartbeat. Tight muscles, rising shoulders, rapid breathing, and clenched fists are also signs of anger.

There are different coping strategies for anger. Let's talk about ten ways to help. You may notice that you may become angry super-fast. I've heard many survivors say that they do not see it coming. Typically, anger strikes an immediate 100 on the scale of 1–10. Even though it surprises you, here are some suggestions given by other brain injury folks. First, if you can, walk away. The best way to keep from saying hurtful things or doing harmful behaviors is to separate from the trigger. Second, bite your tongue. Patti, a TBI survivor, jokingly says that she keeps a bag of tongues with her because she is biting hers off so frequently! I do think there is wisdom in not engaging with someone else when you are angry. So many times, it is not a productive conversation. Third, try changing the subject. You may want to tell your loved ones to help you by changing the subject. It helps you think about something else, which reduces the anger and helps you focus on something that is not triggering. Fourth, after you have calmed down, talk to your loved one about the incident. See if you both can create a plan of action next time you are triggered. Fifth, apologize if you have said or done something offensive. It is good to take responsibility for one's behavior, even if it is humbling. Saying something like, "my bad" or "I'm sorry" or "I messed up" shows the other person that you are aware of the wrong and being accountable. Sixth, if you have the awareness that you are becoming angry, tell someone. Perhaps the person can remind you of some of the strategies that may help lessen or alleviate anger. Seventh, consider playing music to settle down. One of our young survivors says that when he gets upset or angry, he retreats to his room and listens to his favorite music. He says that inevitably he feels better. Eighth, practice mindfulness. That means focusing on what is happening now. Tune your senses into your environment. What are you seeing? What are you hearing? What is the room temperature? What is happening in your body? Focus on your breathing. Deep breaths can help you relax. It will also help you meditate on something positive. Ninth, exercise may help. Sometimes punching a pillow is a non-harmful exercise. Some choose to walk to release anger. A physical activity can help transition anger energy into creativity without hurting yourself or someone else. Tenth, practice relaxation techniques. This includes progressive muscle relaxation. Sometimes it helps to use imagery like floating on a cloud (see appendix A, "Visualization – Cloud"). Consider researching what relaxation scripts fit you and your personality. Have those on hand for times of anger. Choose the strategy that most suits you.

About medication…please ask your provider if anger or agitation is a side effect of any of your medication. For example, some survivors have found that some drugs for seizures make them more agitated and generally irritable. Also, there are medications that can help stabilize your moods and reduce the anger outbursts. Consider asking your physiatrist or brain injury medical provider about a prescription found to help with mood swings.

Here are a few other coping strategies that may help with anger:

1. Creating and keeping a consistent schedule will help avoid some of the unexpected changes. You may consider having a calendar that lists all your appointments and chores for the day. Routine and structure help you know what to expect and what to plan for and reduce frustration.
2. Create a calm environment. Minimize noise and distractions. Create a quiet and peaceful room or setting. One of my friends has a corner in her bedroom that is only used for journaling and meditation. Her family knows that when she is in her chair in her room, they are not to disturb her.
3. Give yourself grace. So many times, I have seen survivors be hard on themselves when they mess up or make a mistake. Especially, those who were go-getters before the injury tend to be very hard on themselves if they have to go at a slower pace towards healing. Please know that you are getting better. Add grace to your pace. When you do, life will get easier for you.
4. Develop a hobby. One of my survivor friends just told me that she has started working on jigsaw puzzles. She was so excited to tell me she had completed two! As you know, the dexterity, patience, and problem-solving that puzzles require help speed the cognitive process. Hobbies can also give you a positive outlet for your emotions. They help you to concentrate on something productive and creative to enjoy.
5. Take naps or breaks. Adequate rest reduces the fatigue that makes anger and irritability worse. If you cannot sleep, try safely closing your eyes for 20 or 30 seconds. Closing your eyes helps preserve approximately 40 percent of your brain's energy! This is a handy trick when in public and the environment overwhelms you. Ensure you are safe and then "rest your eyes" for a few seconds.

By combining these techniques, you and your caregiver can manage your anger and improve your emotional stability. With a TBI, it takes a long time for the brain to heal. The anger flare-ups can be more indicative of such things as a fatigue/migraine combination. So, with both of those issues, rest and quiet are a helpful way to manage them. And when you have an outburst, it is good for you to go back and apologize in your own time and in your own pace. I know that it's hard. Just like you are learning to pace your cognitive work, you have to pace your emotional and physical work too. Sometimes that's hard to do when you have so many demands on you.

One of the most effective resources available to you are support groups. Nowadays you can participate in person or online, especially when you live outside a major metroplex. In the support group you will find others who struggle with anger just as you do. Some have been able to utilize coping skills that have helped them deal with the outbursts in a healthier fashion. Support groups also help you not feel so alone. Brain injury tends to isolate, doesn't it? Most people in your life do not have a brain injury and do not understand what you are going through. You may encourage your caregiver to do the same. There are support groups for caregivers of TBI survivors. One of the aspects that I appreciate is that most participants are in different stages of brain injury recovery. So, it is likely that someone has already traveled the road you are on. Various social media outlets have groups to join. There are also brain injury rehabilitation programs that offer peer support. You may research what is available in your area.

Because you are reading this book, you are already open to knowing more about counseling. I have found that individual and family therapy is a crucial part of recovery. As you know, most TBI folks and family members are initially focused on survival. As time goes by, it becomes clearer that there are and will be a variety of changes. The stages of healing have their own challenges. Unfortunately, outpatient counseling (as of this writing) is not always the first thing people consider. However, this allows you to have an objective listener, someone well-versed in brain injury and mental health who can join forces in helping you and the caregiver overcome these challenges and reintegrate into the community. I recommend that the survivor and caregiver have separate time with the therapist. On occasion it will be beneficial to have a joint session. The therapy may focus on loss, depression, anxiety, and/or transitioning back to family, social, and work life. The technique that research says is most effective with brain injury is cognitive-behavioral therapy (CBT). This technique helps you understand how your thoughts contribute to your feelings and your behavior. Basically, this approach helps you recognize negative thoughts or beliefs. One that I hear often is, "I will never get better." Thanks to neuroplasticity, you will always be improving! See how changing that negative thought to a hopeful truth can give you hope? That's just one example. In my dissertation, I asked survivors and caregivers what their greatest needs were. The survivors said that they needed (1) patience and (2) understanding. The caregivers said that they needed (1) understanding and (2) patience. In my years of practice, I have realized that this finding is true. Patience in the healing process and understanding of what brain injury is, what it means, and how it affects each person. Therapy and psychoeducation (learning about the various aspects of brain injury and mental health) can provide both needs.

One of the ways you can manage the emotional output is to have a regular outlet such as journaling or screaming into a pillow or another non-harmful activity. You have a lot to be angry about and now that you are dealing with the tragic trauma, you may have more mini-explosions. Think of letting air out of a balloon. Expressing anger in healthy ways keeps one from exploding. Try to come up with ways you can express anger, sadness, and frustration in small ways during the day. I think that will keep you from exploding on someone unaware. Anger is a God-given emotion that is protective in nature and needed to remedy mistreatment. Be curious about it. What is it telling you? How can you use the energy from anger to heal?

Believe it or not, you are getting healthier emotionally. It feels rotten, but it is very healthy to be angry. So, there are three types of anger. The most severe is depression/shutdown. The second level is being generally mad at everyone. This is better than depression but not exactly good. The healthiest expression of anger is directing it towards the person who offended you. Remember that normally you are not an angry person. You are a wounded person. Embrace her; comfort her; let her be mad; go get ice cream (do something fun).

So, remember, anger can be a healthy emotion meant to help you know something is off. Anger is not wrong. In fact, God calls us to be angry. Check out what the apostle Paul says in Ephesians 4:26: "Be angry and do not sin; do not let the sun go down on your anger" (English Standard Version). Righteous anger comes from God. We are to use its energy constructively when something wrong has happened. Try using some of the techniques and information given here. Oh, let me add one more technique. It comes from Proverbs 15:1 which says, "A soft answer turns away wrath, but a harsh word stirs up anger" (ESV). Try your best to respond with gentleness. I know that's super-hard but give it a go. It takes discipline but is well worth the effort. When one allows for the anger, places it appropriately, then one can experience a new kind of joy. This joy is what is coming for you. In fact, you may have experienced bubbles of it already!

Until next time,
Deana

Homework

- Create a plan to use when you are angry.

_____

_____

- Investigate what anger is telling you. How is it a map to the current situation? What happened before the anger episode? Did someone hurt your feelings? Are you fatigued?

_____

_____

Resources

Edward, L. (2023). *Anger management after brain injury: Understanding anger after TBI, mTBI or concussion care guide.* ISBNservices.com.

Newark, A., & Roy-Bornstein, C. (2014). *Chicken soup for the soul: Recovering from traumatic brain injuries.* Chicken Soup for the Soul.

7 Relationships

In chapter 3, "Family Experience of a Loved One with Brain Injury", I primarily addressed the family experience after a brain injury. In this chapter, we will focus specifically on the different types of relationships (spouses, parents, children, friends, colleagues, acquaintances, and siblings) that are affected by brain injury. Certainly, it is a challenge to understand how you fit into the family and what roles and responsibilities you have after brain injury. It is especially difficult when you are not sure who you are post-injury! For example, Rich felt bad because he used to be the breadwinner of the family. After his injury, he was not able to work. What role does he have as a husband and father now? So, let's look at specific relationships. How have the roles changed? What are the expectations? What is a healthy relationship? How do we create an environment of change and acceptance? What is healthy communication? Let's dive in!

Partners

One of the most researched relationships of brain injury families is the partner or spouse relationship. Depending on the researcher, separation and divorce are higher in couples when one partner has a TBI. Other researchers say that the rate is lower than in the normal population. From my experience, divorces tend to be more common than in the non-head-injured relationships. I believe this has to do with the health of the marriage before the injury. Observing couples for the last several years, those with a splintering marriage before the injury normally do not adjust well to the injury. From my experience, the relationship carries similar behaviors post-injury as they had pre-injury. For example, Sarah intended to divorce her husband but when he had the accident, she did not believe she could divorce him. Her reasoning was that "it looks bad" for me to divorce someone with a disability.

DOI: 10.4324/9781003602774-7

She remained in the marriage for three years post-accident but then did go ahead and divorced him. If the couple were in a healthy relationship before the accident or injury and then divorced, I think it is because the non-injured spouse chooses not to know about TBI or does not want to be responsible for the outcome of someone who is injured. I've also found that a few couples get married with full knowledge that one partner has a TBI. And although the non-injured partner has limited information about how TBI affects her husband, the commitment is there to learn, support, and encourage. Love, loyalty, understanding, and kindness towards each other determine how well they navigate the brain injury challenges. In many ways the person they married is not the person they are now. They have to get to know one another again like when they first dated. So, it is essential for non-injured partners to become educated about brain injury. Read books about brain injury. Talk to other brain injury survivors and their care partners. Certainly, working with a couple's counselor is suggested to help couples navigate the catastrophic results and changes in their relationship. It is important for the counselor to be well-versed in working with TBI. My suggestion for any therapist is to educate herself in all aspects and in the developmental stages of recovery. If they can understand the factors of brain injury from the onset of the injury through reintegration into the community, they will be much more effective as a counselor. Plus, the counselor will be able to recognize a deficit of brain injury versus a mental health issue versus a character issue. Without the training, she can misdiagnose and misunderstand an issue. For example, when a husband with TBI does not remember to buy something at the store, it is not because he wasn't listening or doesn't care. It is because his short-term memory is damaged. Knowing something has an organic root (the brain injury) helps their spouses not take the mistakes personally and extend more grace to their partner.

You may have noticed that communication style changes with brain injury. Depending on the severity and type of head injury, communication can have a whole other cadence or flow. In other words, your loved one may not be able to communicate with you as before. Brain injury causes slower processing of conversation and a change in perception. Therefore, it is wise to communicate with your spouse in a slower (not condescending) pattern. Here are a few other changes to consider. Again, these are generalizations and may not apply to every situation.

1. Because there is slower processing, adjust your rate of speech. In other words, talking at a fast speed can frustrate your partner who is trying his best to follow you but can't. Slow down.

Pronounce the consonants. Stay on the same topic. Check for understanding before moving to another topic.
2. Because there are short-term memory issues, be OK with reminding your loved one of an appointment or chore or activity. It is helpful to have a sticky note or a whiteboard to write down what needs to be remembered that part of the day, week, or month. When shopping, make a list of items to purchase.
3. Because there is limited abstract thought, relate concretely. Think about concrete as something that can be seen, touched, or heard. Abstract concepts are things that cannot be perceived through the senses. Be specific. One of the couples particularly struggled with this because the wife would say, "Henry, will you please go to the store and get garden fencing?" The request is too broad. He went to the store but brought back several different fencing items that she didn't want. Sherry needed to be specific.
4. Because fatigue is a large part of the recovery process, allow your spouse to rest. If he says that he is too tired to do something, believe him. Please consider adjusting the schedule to accommodate his energy level. Mornings are typically better for cognitively challenging activities.
5. Because irritation may be part of the recovery process, do your best not to take statements personally. Sometimes it is simply the frustration coming out, not a personal attack. If your spouse is angry, give him space to be alone and calm down. Arguing makes the situation worse.
6. Because his sense of humor may have changed, be prepared for a more childlike or juvenile humor (at times) that seems silly and immature.
7. Because your partner may have limited insight into his social behavior, consider working together to create a sign that both of you know that signals he is talking too much or interrupting. Victor lightly touches his wife's hand when she is going on and on about a topic. Her TBI made it difficult for her to recognize the social cues that signal a topic change. The give and take (each person taking turns talking) in conversation need to be relearned. Sometimes the survivor does not recognize the social cues for changing the subject, ending a conversation, etc.
8. Because marital roles have likely changed with brain injury, share with one another expectations of the current roles. As recovery continues, the roles may continue to change. Being able to navigate those changes is important. The survivor may be able to take on more responsibility and participate as a partner. For example,

before the accident Hugh's role was to clean up after dinner. After his TBI, he was unable to clean up because he was too fatigued to wash dishes etc. So, he and his wife adjusted their expectations and responsibilities to fit what he was able to do, which was set the table.

9. Because nonverbal communication is their first language, be mindful of your body language, tone of voice, facial expression, and gestures. Generally, nonverbal communication is about 93% of communication and the words we use are only 7%. Often when there is a misunderstanding it is due to the words not matching the body language. Patti, a TBI survivor, says it like this: "Make sure your audio matches your video." What I have noticed is that sometimes when there is a disagreement, it is because the survivor is reading the nonverbal message instead of listening to the words. In my opinion, it will serve the relationship well if the spouse is mindful of how she is coming across as much as what she is saying. Communication works most effectively when the nonverbal and verbal interactions convey the same message.

10. Because the survivor may have new personality traits, it is possible that the spouse may feel like she is "married to a stranger". Personality changes call for each partner to be patient and get to know one another again like when the relationship originally began. When people get to know one another, it takes time to understand and learn who they are. The challenge is in expecting the person who looks the same to act the same. Shelly, the wife of Tom, a TBI survivor, said that she tries to not compare Tom with who he was because, "It isn't fair to make someone live in the shadow of someone they are not." A huge statement indeed!

Briefly, the sexual relationship may have also changed with brain injury. Sometimes the survivor experiences greater sexual desire or sometimes it is decreased. Research says that at least half of brain injury survivors experience decreased sex drive. If the sexual desire has increased there is a possibility of inappropriate behavior or comments. This is most often seen in transitional rehabilitation programs. A possible reason for the increased sexual drive or activity is due to damage in the frontal lobe. This area helps control impulses and social inhibitions. Privately, communicate with your partner that the behavior can be seen as offensive and why. Healthy communication is needed to help both partners work through the changes in intimacy. Consider correcting the behavior in a kind manner and not shaming the survivor. Sexual arousal may also be affected so that it is hard for the body to respond to stimulation. The difficulty may be due to hormone changes, self-confidence, as well as increased stress in the relationship. It may be helpful for a man to discuss the sexual activity or feelings with another man. Or for a woman to speak to another woman. These challenges are normal for couples dealing with brain injury. Communicate with one another about how to navigate the changes and, if needed, seek a counselor who understands brain injury and the role of sexual intimacy in relationships.

As we mentioned earlier in this chapter, a major stressor in relationships is the changes of roles and responsibilities. The severity of the brain injury determines the extent of those changes. Also, the trajectory (direction and rate) of recovery dictates how the roles and responsibilities alter from time to time. For example, at the beginning of the recovery process, the survivor may not be able to participate in activities of daily living like getting ready for the day. However, as he continues in therapy (occupational/physical/speech) he can do more for himself. A complication is that the ability of the survivor may change from day to day. So, it is important to expect the inconsistency rather than assume that he can function at the same level every day. Megan, the wife of Steve, adjusted her expectations according to his fatigue level. So, if he felt more energy, he could help pick up the kids from school. If he was fatigued, she would make other arrangements. Although the constant change was challenging, they were able to communicate and help each other with what to expect.

Parenting

TBI affects the whole family. And when your survivor looks the same as he did before the accident, it is hard to remember he has a brain injury. As a parent with TBI, raising a family and keeping the household running can be extremely challenging. As wonderful as children are, they need directions on how to best support the parent with brain injury. They also need someone to talk to about the changes they experience or notice in their dad, for example. Good communication, love, understanding, and attention are helpful in creating a happy, healthy family. If possible, consistent co-parenting with your spouse eases some of the burden of responsibilities. The age of the children affects the adjustments needed in a parenting relationship. Teenagers tend to naturally assume more responsibility than toddlers. Robert's children were only five and six when he was injured in a car wreck. His wife, Carol, was great about helping them adjust to their dad. Although it was very challenging for Carol, she was able to organize and plan to accommodate Robert's brain injury and help the kids know how to communicate with their dad. One of the things she did was plan for all of them to watch one of the kids' favorite shows. Robert (because he was early in recovery) also enjoyed the same shows. It was as though he was one of the kids. This isn't an insult as much as an observation that those with severe TBI can enjoy children's shows because they are easier to track and understand, thereby causing less brain fatigue and overload. Adult movies and shows tend to have embedded messaging that is hard to track.

Part of good communication is creating visible reminders of appointments and chores. Many families have a whiteboard located in the kitchen that lists all of the activities of each member of the family. Consider color coding so that at a glance, you can see that the activity is for Robert (red) or Carol (blue) or one of the children (yellow or green). Sonya took the opportunity to teach her children about how to take care of their dad who was in a wheelchair. She adjusted their responsibilities according to their age and ability. Sonya said that she believed that her children became more intuitive about struggles others have. She mentioned that they are kinder and less afraid to talk to someone with a disability. Sonya and her husband were open with their children about what had happened to their dad and how it had affected him. Keeping the door of communication open helped the children discuss what they didn't understand or what may scare them. Creating a safety plan in case of a crisis is another way of calming and educating the children in case of an emergency. For example, make a list of people to call such as emergency services, a neighbor, or a trusted family member.

A deficit of brain injury that could negatively affect the family dynamic is irritability and agitation, which often happens as the brain heals. And the agitation is more apt when the survivor is fatigued. It has been suggested by other survivors that when you become agitated, put yourself in a time-out. In other words, separate oneself from the family to help calm down. James admitted that he has a shorter fuse when it comes to discipline. He recognized that he gets agitated quicker at night than during the day. Fatigue played a big role in how he managed his anger. He and his wife told their sons to be more mindful to do what dad asked quicker than later. It is part of accommodating emotional outbursts. Sometimes James would ask his wife to take over whatever task they were working on so he could remove himself and calm down. Losing one's temper or being easily agitated can be a part of early recovery as well as a long-term deficit depending on where the brain injury is. It is important to educate the family that the agitation is a result of the injury and not a character problem of the survivor. Typically, kids manage the deficits of a parent with brain injury if they are informed and given instructions about what to do when they manifest. Working with a counselor who understands brain injury is also a helpful strategy for the family. Sarah advised her kids to leave their dad alone and do something else in a different room. This strategy, she said, helped her husband calm down and eventually join the family. She said that he also apologizes to the kids if he says something hurtful. Older children have similar confusion on how to manage the emotions of the injured parent. Richard has 4 daughters who were from age 16 to 24 when he was injured. The older children took time away from college and work to attend to their dad. Although the initial reaction was fear and confusion, as Richard recovered, they began to feel depressed and anxious about what their future as a family may look like. Their mom helped them understand what brain injury is and what to expect as far as they knew. She also directed the girls to concentrate on their schooling when not helping the family. Three years after the injury, all the daughters have a unique relationship with their dad whereby they offer support as he needs. Richard is good at expressing appreciation of their help but quick to encourage them to get on with their lives, which they have done.

Siblings

Having a brother or sister that has experienced a brain injury is very challenging for the family. Siblings have a variety of feelings associated with injury ranging from anger, depression, fear, and confusion to jealousy and guilt. This tends to happen when the parents and extended family focus on the injured sibling. Siblings can feel left out and unimportant in these situations. The family dynamics before the injury affect how the family unit reacts to the survivor and one another. Meaning, if a family has open communication and healthy attitudes towards one another, they will most likely act similarly in response to a chaotic event. However, it can be difficult to make sense of the situation and their own feelings about what happened. Sadly, because of the severity of the injury, siblings can be forgotten victims. Certainly, it is not intentional, but it is normal when the resources of the family must be directed at someone's survival. Of course, educating siblings to the degree they will understand helps reduce confusion and fear. Those are natural reactions that come with a catastrophic incident. Encourage the siblings to visit and participate in rehabilitation as much as they are comfortable. This will help build trust in the relationship. As the survivor gets better, they can discover new activities that they can do together. Doing relaxing activities is also encouraged. Walking or sitting in a park can be helpful in getting to know one another again in a less stressful way. One of the most difficult issues is when the survivor does not act the same as before the injury. This is particularly hard if he looks the same. It is important to remind the siblings not to take it personally if the survivor says something off-color or out of line. Give siblings their own time to talk to someone where they can say and process their feelings about their survivor. Counseling and/or support groups are great spaces for them to process feeling jealous or guilty or depressed or relieved. There are so many emotions that come to the forefront depending on the recovery of the survivor and how the family deals with the incident. Participating in support groups can also build confidence in the survivor because he will be with others who understand some of his struggles.

If the siblings are adults, the brother or sister often becomes responsible for the survivor. They may become their guardian and/or durable power of attorney and/or medical power of attorney. This may also include being responsible for the survivor's financial and medical expenses and commitments. In these circumstances, it is wise to consult a legal advisor who is an expert with end-of-life and family estate requirements. Kara, sister of Karl, said that she had taken over caring for her brother when her parents could no longer help him. She said that she is glad that she can help but also feels sad because since his injury, she has been unable to have someone she can relate to. She said that she has become a guardian or parent instead of a sister. She mentioned that this causes her feelings of grief and makes her sad. So, no matter what the sibling's age, it is a challenge to know how to relate to their injured loved one. Support groups are particularly effective in helping siblings not feel alone as they relate to their survivor.

Friendships

A common proverb says, "A friend loves at all times, and a brother is born for adversity" (Proverbs 17:17, English Standard Version). When tragedy hits, friends can become family. In fact, sometimes families are less available than friends. Ruth said that when her daughter was injured, she was surprised at the friends who came to their aid and the family members that did not help. Proverbs 27:9 (The Message) says, "a sweet friendship refreshes the soul." During the initial phase of injury, many family members and friends and acquaintances come to help the family. As the recovery draws on, people tend to fade away while others become more present. It is interesting to see who comes to the forefront and who withdraws. Often it is not who you expect. Marty, a TBI and cancer survivor, said that she was shocked that Kathleen (a friend from 20 years ago) came to be with her during her recovery. She said, "Of all the people I know, I never expected Kathleen to come be with me. What a gift!" It is wonderful to see how friends become family when disaster strikes.

One of the sad outcomes for survivors is the loss of some friends. The reason for this is partially due to the nature of an extended illness. People move on with their lives and become less involved with the family. Of course, this is a source of grief for survivors. However, there is an opportunity to make new friends through common experiences. For example, Craig became friends with Dawson while they both were working out at the same gym. Both were participating in a specialized program for brain injury survivors. Important to creating healthy relationships is talking about brain injury and educating friends about what to expect. Craig and Dawson shared common experiences of dealing with the deficits of brain injury like having a short fuse or not remembering information. They were able to share with their loved ones how to help them when these things happened. As an aside, I recommend families oversee new friendships because survivors tend to be naïve and too trusting. So, a family can protect their loved one from being taken advantage of. This takes time for the survivor to develop good judgement about people and for the family to trust that their survivor can take care of himself.

Colleagues and Acquaintances

Going back to work and community reintegration set the stage for renewed relationships with colleagues and acquaintances. A common question asked by survivors and their families is, "Do I share that I have a brain injury?" The fear is that people may not understand them or judge them unfairly. Makes sense. Sometimes it is helpful to share your story. Other times, it has an adverse effect. For example, Samantha told church members that Rick had a brain injury. She was expecting a kinder, more receptive experience. Instead, people became more distant. It is unfortunate that some respond that way. However, those that lean into the family and want to know more can be a great gift. While doing my dissertation I found that two of the greatest needs for survivors and their families are patience and understanding.

Caregivers needed to be educated about brain injury and needed their family and friends to understand at least partially how it affects the family. Understanding is about education and taking the time to know how brain injury specifically affects the survivor. Survivors need people to be patient with them as they recover. Patience is about extending grace and kindness as the survivor heals. Adjusting expectations to accommodate the recovery process is key to patience and understanding. An example of adjusting expectations is not pushing the survivor to do something they cannot do. Just because the survivor looks the same, it doesn't mean that he is the same. Get to know the new person without expecting him to be who he was before the injury.

Returning to work may mean going back to the same job as before. It can also mean working at a different job that fits their current ability. For example, Ken could not return to his previous work as an electrician, but he could work stocking shelves in an electrical retail store. He still had the knowledge but not the ability to multitask. Some survivors cannot go back to the same job but do work as a volunteer or at a job that better fits their capabilities. After the injury they may need various accommodations such as more time to complete tasks or a quiet environment to work in. Allowing the survivor to return to contributing to society is essential to their finding purpose. And the purpose is a hope lifeline. A lifeline that gives them hope that they can make a difference in their world and that they can make a positive contribution to life. Hal could not return as a plumber but did work part-time as a cashier in a hardware store. He said that it helped him to do something productive and that helps other people. If your loved one desires to return to work, see that as a step of recovery. Do your best to encourage the desire and not discourage the survivor. Vocational rehabilitation counselors can assess the survivor's current ability, and help evaluate what type of job and what type of schedule will accommodate the abilities of the survivor. Vocational counselors normally work with a government agency to help those with disabilities. You may find them at an employment center or at an organization specializing in disabilities.

Letter to You

Dear Community,

As challenging as it may be, walking alongside someone with brain injury is one of the most rewarding experiences you can have. I have found that survivors are this world's testament to resilience. They typically fight to live again and make a difference in their community. They understand at a deep level what it means to fight for their life. What a joy to have the opportunity to share their journey. Walking beside a survivor means putting aside your agenda and expectations. The survivor is the focus, the center stage if you will. It means learning about their abilities and deficits. It means being dedicated to their recovery by attending appointments or having a meal together or sharing their concerns and accomplishments. If you are reading this, you have made the decision to be a friend and journey with a survivor or family member. I'm so thankful! The very people who need advocacy, friendship, and assistance are often without them. Your coming alongside is crucial to their recovery. And guess what? Your life will be richer for it! So, let me share with you some of the strategies that may be beneficial as you journey together. Some of these suggestions may suit and others may not. As I often say, "Eat the meat and spit out the bones." In other words, use what is helpful, dismiss what is not.

1. Remember you are a bigger gift than you realize. Survivors and their families have often been abandoned. Not on purpose but due to others not understanding the nature of brain injury or allowing life to take them away. Embrace the journey. You are a gift, and the journey is a gift.
2. Read, read, read about brain injury. Just like there are no two brain injuries the same, the effects of each brain injury are not the same. However, educating yourself can give you a baseline to understand some of what they are going through. Then, ask them about their individual experience. "Generalize [know brain injury] and customize [know survivor]" is a motto for working with the survivor. Having a basic knowledge of brain injury can help you understand what strategies or resources your survivor may need.
3. Always extend grace. Grace to the survivor, to the family, and to yourself. Trying to cope with brain injury is a hard road. The last thing anyone needs is criticism about how they are recovering or how they are doing something. Encouragement that they can continue to grow and get better is helpful. Grace and gentleness (seasoned with strength) is a winning approach.
4. Celebrate every small step of success. Something as common for normal people as washing your hair is a huge feat for the survivor. If you think about it, he has had to relearn every aspect of living. He must think about doing any task. So, celebrate the "win" of each small step in their recovery.

5 Remember you have no idea what it is like to have a brain injury. Although you may know what it is like to forget something, you do not know what it is like to forget something several times a day. Patti, a TBI survivor, explains it like this: "Brain injury survivors often forget from their gut, not just their mind. This in-the-gut forgetting often causes a desperate sensation or feeling, and even reaction sometimes." It causes a panic in the survivor and makes them wonder what else they have forgotten. It also tends to make them feel stupid, which they are not!

6 Survivors have a slower processor, not lower IQ. (I like to say that survivors are twice as smart as the rest of us because they learned to live from infancy; had brain injury; had to learn to live again. That's twice as smart!) Problem-solving can often take longer. Understanding conversation usually takes longer. Jokes are sometimes harder to "get". So, give your survivor time to think. Don't step on their silence. Be mindful of your speed of speech. Try not to jump topics quickly because he may want to contribute to the conversation. Perhaps check in with the survivor by asking a specific question like, "Tell me something about your morning." Or, "How's your balance today?" Then let the survivor answer at his pace. Sometimes he may talk more than you expected.

7 Allow for the inconsistencies of recovery. Just because the survivor functions well one day (or parts of a day like breakfast or lunch) does not mean he will function well the next day. As the brain heals, the pace of recovery changes from day to day. It is more accurate to compare progress from the day of the injury to the current time instead of comparing the injured person to their pre-injury self. This isn't fair to them.

8 Laugh with them. This helps when the survivor may feel embarrassed. Elizabeth said that it helps her to laugh at herself when she makes a mistake. It just means she is trying.

9 Do not tell the survivor what to do. Since they are trying to use their brain, try not to get in the way by telling them what to do. Instead, try encouraging their decision. Second-guessing can be a part of the recovery process. So, it is more helpful to affirm a good decision. You may offer suggestions if the survivor is open to it.

10 Be mindful of correcting too much. In brain injury recovery, some survivors use confabulation, which happens when they can remember the beginning of a story and the end of a story but not the middle. So, they make the middle up. It is a lie, but it is not meant to deceive but rather to make sense of the rest. In normal relationships, the tendency is to correct one another if someone

misspoke. The issue is that too much correcting can have a shaming effect. There are some things that need correction such as upcoming appointments. But, there are other things that do not require correction. For example, if a survivor says that he had pancakes for breakfast, but he really had cereal, does that really need correcting? No. In the grand scheme of things, what he ate for breakfast is not a big deal and therefore does not require correction. Figuring out what needs correction is a process. However, choosing not to correct every little thing will help avoid conflict and hurt feelings. If the survivor corrects himself, cheer him on and celebrate it!

11 Encourage the survivor to create routines. It is easier on the survivor if he knows what to expect and when. Routine is easier on the brain. Our friend Patti, a TBI survivor, says that, "Consistency serves as a strong, unspoken reminder that helps them learn to cope with short-term memory problems." Schedule activities for the same day at the same time (as much as possible). For example, laundry can be scheduled for Monday mornings. As a counselor, my survivors have the same appointment day and time each week. I try not to vary their schedule. Changing schedules may add extra stress on the survivor because he has to pivot the plan, which can be difficult. Some survivors may "freeze" or "stall out" when there has been an abrupt change. Meaning, he cannot think about an alternative plan. Robert had lunch plans with a friend. The friend cancelled the lunch while Robert was en route. He called and said he didn't know what to do. I responded, "Robert, it's going to be OK. Just turn around and go home." That simple direction helped him because the change had created a crisis for him. Now, this is not always the case, but it is important to be mindful of the possibility.

12 Be prepared to repeat yourself. Sometimes the survivor needs you to write down things. Sometimes, they may need you to repeat yourself. Please do not take the need for repeating yourself personally. Try not to talk down to them or have a condescending tone or expression. Sometimes rephrasing comments or questions can help with understanding. Short-term memory loss is a very common deficit with brain injury. So, that means, more often than not, you will have to remind the survivor of an event or situation, or request.

Homework

- List four things you would want a new friend to know about you.

_____

_____

_____

_____

- List two things that make a good friend to you. For example, someone who makes you laugh or someone who likes the same things you like.

_____

_____

- List two relationships that have especially encouraged you after your brain injury.

_____

_____

- List two things that you learned about relationships since your brain injury.

_____

_____

Resources

Foster, P. (2021). *The adventures of Head Trauma Hero.* Redemption Press.
Senelick, R. (2013). *Living with brain injury: A guide for patients and families* (3rd ed.). Healthsouth Press.
Crimmins, C. (2001). *Where is the mango princess? A journey back from brain injury.* Knopf Doubleday Publishing Group.
Morgan, C. (2010). *The stranger in our marriage: A partner's guide to navigating traumatic brain injury.* Peppertree Press.

8 Grief and Ambiguous Loss

Grieving

Grief is both a painful and an essential part of recovery. Grief is messy. Processing grief means navigating a new life and freedom while honoring the loss of a loved one or past life. When one experiences loss, whether of a person or a lifestyle, the transition does not sail smoothly through Kübler-Ross' five stages of grief (denial, anger, bargaining, depression, acceptance). More typically, one bounces from one stage to the other in no set order. Sometimes one can experience all five stages within a short period of time! Meaning, in one day you can be in denial or shock, and then move to anger and then to acceptance and back to denial. That is why I say that grief is messy. There is also ambiguous loss, which is loss of a culture, experience, vision, idea. Simply, an ambiguous thing is something you feel but cannot see. It is something that is both present and absent at the same time. Pauline Boss (2010) formally identifies two types of ambiguous loss. Type One occurs when someone is physically absent but psychologically present. Examples of this type are missing bodies due to tsunamis or other natural disasters, divorce, adoption, or alienation from family members. Type Two occurs when there is a psychological absence (emotionally or cognitively gone or missing) with a physical presence. Examples of this type are people with traumatic brain injury (TBI), dementia, or addiction. This could also be a preoccupation with losses that do not make sense, such as suicide. I've noticed throughout my work with caregivers and survivors that they may experience both the grief of losing a loved one and ambiguous loss of losing a lifestyle. For example, Tanya's husband died in the same car wreck that caused her TBI. She was not told about his death immediately because she was unable to process it. Plus, the medical team did not want her to know because the news might have adversely affected her desire to get better and recover. After several weeks, she was told that he had not made it through the wreck. They also reassured her that it was not her fault that he died. Initially, she said that she couldn't believe it and thought that people were lying to her. Then, she was angry that he died. Her own brain injury made it difficult for her to process his death. After jumping to the various stages of grief, she realized that he was gone. She said that she was relieved that he did not suffer or see her injured. Because the date of death and the date she was told were different, she grieved her husband's death on the day she found out about it. So, for her, she had the experience of losing a person (grief) and losing a life with her beloved husband (ambiguous loss).

Elisabeth Kübler-Ross (1969) explains the grief stages as follows: (a) denial, (b) anger, (c) bargaining, (d) depression, and (e) acceptance. Denial is the initial reaction when one learns of a death. Considered a temporary defense, the individual may not believe that his/her loved one has died. Harold Elliott, a police chaplain, specialized in death notifications. He said that when he tells a loved one of a death, he is very clear because during the initial stage softer language is often misunderstood. So, he will say, "Mr. Smith, your wife, Alice, is dead." Harold told me in a private conversation that it is important to not use words like, "expired, passed away, lost" because often the receiver will misunderstand. While it may seem harsh, a direct approach saves more confusion in an already chaotic time. The second stage, anger, happens when denial no longer works. Anger is often misdirected to someone who is not responsible for their loved one's death. It can be directed inwardly as well. Blaming themselves is part of anger and the bargaining stage. Questions such as, "Why me?" or, "Why did this happen?" are common. Bargaining occurs when one hopes that s/he can change the outcome. Typically, people will try to negotiate with God or try to bargain for a more acceptable alternative besides death. For example, if this had not happened then my loved one would not have died. Depression is the stage where the reality of the death sets in. Emptiness and loneliness become silent partners for the survivor. The person with grief-associated depression prefers to isolate and be silent. While being alone can be helpful, talking to a trusted friend or participating in a grief support group will offer coping strategies to deal with the feelings. Acceptance means coming to terms with the fact that your loved one has died. It incorporates the hope of a future. Navigating these stages is different for everyone. Some want to be alone. Others want to travel. Still others want to investigate all the details surrounding the death of a loved one. The various reactions relate to one's disposition, the type of death, cultural mores, one's support system, and the kind of relationship one had with the person who died. Culture traditions may help the person process death. Funeral traditions vary in different parts of the world. For example, Tibet and Mongolia practice sky burial where the body is left exposed to the elements. China hangs coffins in hard-to-get-to places such as mountainsides. Nordic countries practice water burials while aboriginal societies perform smoking ceremonies.

From a Survivor's Perspective

I have found that the experience of brain injury lends itself to a multitude of losses, most of which would fall into the category of ambiguous loss. Think about the changes in work life, family life, and social life. The routine of getting up to go to work, going to work, and coming home has all changed. Patti, a TBI survivor, said that she had to relearn every function of living. Interestingly, when her family had asked her about her job, she did not know what a job was, much less that she had to have one. It took time for her to remember that she was a speaker and a famous radio personality. Part of her rehabilitation incorporated her previous speaking skills. She was given an opportunity to speak in front of fellow patients. Her medical team wanted her to have an opportunity to give a speech since she had been a motivational speaker before the wreck. So, Patti experienced the ambiguous losses of routine, of work, of earning a living, etc. Some survivors can return to their previous occupation, but many cannot. Part of the recovery process is helping survivors recognize their strengths and desires. It may mean returning to the same work, but often it means working at a different job and at a different pace. Patti returned to motivational (inspirational) speaking but did not return to being a radio personality. For work, the survivor participates in various therapy sessions. Their routine is going from appointment to appointment. I often tell my clients that their work is getting better and doing the activities and treatments recommended to them. Just as we would not expect a toddler to drive, we cannot expect a survivor to perform greater than their current ability. We can anticipate growth and improvement in due course. It is helpful to allow for the adjustment and embrace the new experiences instead of feeling negative about the slowed pace. This will help the survivor find purpose, which we will talk more about in the last chapter. But for now, suffice it to say, lack of purpose seems to be one of the most difficult losses to overcome. And once overcome, purpose gives meaning to all the suffering since the brain injury.

How long does grief last? The research says that the normal grief period is approximately one to two years. But that is a generalization. The sense of yearning can last a lifetime. Yearning is an intense longing that can occur throughout the grieving process. It is normal to pine for your loved one. It is normal to yearn to be who you used to be. If we don't grieve, it means we don't love. It is another way to express one's love for a person or situation. Hopefully, in time, one's experience of grief will lessen. Not because your love for the person has diminished, but because life has become bigger. It's about width, not depth. The intensity of one's feelings lessens as time goes on although the anniversary of the death or special occasions may trigger a fresh wave of grief. Again, this is normal. What is not normal is when someone feels the intensity of initial grief several years down the road. Rachel, a TBI survivor, lost her daughter to suicide. Ten years after her daughter's death, Rachel had not touched her daughter's room. It remained the same as on the day she died. This is a complicated grief reaction. In Rachel's case, her grief was frozen in time just like the room. Perhaps you are having trouble reintegrating back into life or still experiencing deep emotional pain (anger, bitterness, sorrow) or intense loneliness. This would be considered complicated grief or prolonged grief. If that is the case, professional help is warranted.

From a Caregiver's Perspective

Grief and ambiguous loss associated with brain injury are difficult to manage. Family members, friends, and colleagues all experience the loss of the function of the TBI survivor as well as the enormous change in family life and the social system. Relationship shifts, changes in friendships, and strain on family life are a few of the issues associated with ambiguous loss that accompany brain injury. Family members continue to wait for the pre-injury person to reappear, like they are a broken arm. With enough therapy and treatment the arm will return to normal. Unfortunately, the brain injury survivor seldom returns to "normal". When the caregiver realizes that their TBI survivor will not return to his pre-injury self, they experience the anger stage of loss. Connecting with a support group of fellow caregivers will help process this difficult stage of grief. Counseling with a therapist well-versed in brain injury, grief, and ambiguous loss will also assist in dealing with the variants of brain injury losses.

Another loss is the social and family system changes. Friends and family react differently to the survivor. Some are great at visiting and want to know about TBI. Others are waiting for the survivor to return to normal. When that doesn't happen, they move on with their lives and away from the survivor. Unfortunately, friends tend to fade away after the initial injury. Most everyone is attentive during the initial injury. But over time, people get on with their lives and spend less time with the TBI survivor. While that is normal, it is also painful and disheartening. Along with the fading of friends, some family members leave. They do so in the form of denial or becoming less available to help. I've seen this in my practice. Family members are very supportive and attentive during the initial crisis but become less available the longer the recovery lasts. Some extended families choose to blame the victim or the medical system or the caregiver for the recovery not being fast enough. This is tragic and counter to most brain injury recovery. Due to the nature of TBI, healing is a slow process. It is not the six-week recovery time of a broken bone. The brain must recreate neural pathways, which take time. Sadly, some families deny the long-term effects of brain injury and choose not to learn about TBI. One may hear comments such as, "She is faking" or, "He looks fine." Not being believed or having the TBI acknowledged adds to the grief. Certainly, the loss of function, the loss of relationships, and the loss of dreams and purpose are also examples of ambiguous losses specific to brain injury. This is another chance for caregivers to participate in a support group. Other caregivers have most likely already traveled the recovery road that you are on and have suggestions to help you navigate the grief terrain.

Caregiver grief is another aspect of loss associated with brain injury. Often caregivers experience the loss of the personality of the loved one who was injured. As mentioned earlier, they wait for the pre-injury person to return so when it does not happen, they feel sadness, guilt, anger, and frustration. Longing for the pre-injury loved one is normal. It is a part of the process of ambiguous loss. Pauline Boss (2010) explained that ambiguous loss is a state that does not provide finality. What I have found in working with survivors is that the ambiguous losses seem to be more complicated to manage than actual death. In fact, some have even commented that death would have been easier. I believe this is because ambiguous loss does not offer formal closure such as a funeral or a wake. It feels perpetual. For example, the survivor or caregiver will experience new and ongoing losses such as an inability to drive or hold a full-time job. Also, when the time markers or milestones of development are missed, the survivor feels additional loss. What I mean is that sometimes the survivor is given the expectation that they will be better in a month or a year. This is not always realistic. Yes, there are improvements but not total recovery. So, when one month or one year passes without full recovery, the survivor feels deflated, guilty, angry, and/or scared. They feel the loss of not meeting a time expectation. Recovery is a complicated dance between recognizing loss and embracing gains. These are a sample of hundreds of examples. So, let me address these concerns in my letter about grief and ambiguous loss.

Letter to You

Dear Friend,

Grief is messy. Not only does it not move smoothly through the five stages of grief (denial, anger, bargaining, depression, acceptance); it also collects all the losses from the past and mixes it up with the present.... a mess indeed! So don't be surprised if you are thinking again and grieving again about people who have died in the past. It is not that you haven't dealt with the losses before, they just move to the "front and center" of your brain again. This is the nature of grief. Also, one can experience all the five stages within a few minutes! So, what do you do? Well, recognize it for what it is. Grief is a tribute to your love. It is a place to honor your loved one and your past. Honor your tears. King David would pray, "Lord, you keep track of all my sorrows. You have collected all my tears in your bottle. You have recorded each one in your book" (Psalm 56:8, New Living Translation). My interpretation: "Lord, take what's precious to me and cherish them." Tears are the language of the heart. Embrace them. It's OK to let them express what you can't put into words. Research says that tears expressed with another person have more healing properties than tears shed alone. So, share your grief with someone you trust.

The depression stage of grief is the internal voice that says negative things about yourself and the future. It's not you, per se. Depression tends to have a "doom and gloom" voice. It's not always the truth. So do your best to acknowledge the loss and the depression. Recognize it as a current stage, not a permanent state. Anger or irritability may accompany depression. I was given a wonderful piece of advice by Rosa, my Holocaust and TBI survivor friend. Her family was killed in the gas chambers in Auschwitz. She told me (after my mother-in-law died), "If your husband is cross [her word for irritable], don't hear it. That is grief talking." That advice has served me well. And I believe it will serve you too. It is so helpful to not take the irritable comments personally. It saves a lot of heartache and argument. But if you have been experiencing depression for several weeks, please contact your doctor. And of course, if you feel like you are a danger to yourself or others, call emergency services.

Years ago, Judith Viorst wrote *Necessary Losses*. This is a book about all the losses that come with change and growth. I believe that is something you are dealing with...the losses associated with recovery. If you think about it, nothing is the same after a catastrophic event. Even if things look similar, they are different. Sort of like a book with the same cover but different content. It takes time to process all the losses associated with a brain injury. Your family is experiencing similar grief. However, they are experiencing it from an external perspective while you are experiencing it both internally and externally. In other words, you know more fully what you have lost and are dealing with while they have a different perspective. What I see often is that the survivor and their loved one tend to compare the present self with the pre-injury self. Honestly, I think that is part of the denial. It is easier to expect a full return to pre-injury health than recognize there are major changes. Do your best not to entertain that kind of thinking. It makes the grieving worse and is not at all accurate. The fairest comparison is between the day of the injury and today. In other words, do not compare your current self with yourself before the injury. That's not helpful. Instead, compare your current self with the day you were injured. You will be able to see vast changes and improvement! When you can see the growth, it helps with mitigating the grief. And remember, grief is a doorway, not a dead end or full stop.

Maybe you've said, "That person died" when talking about your pre-injury self. That is a huge statement. It means that you are acknowledging that loss! Take the time you need to recognize what those losses mean. Cry, scream, or pound a pillow to release some of those emotions. You have a right to them. Yes, you are different. Yes. However, you are not diminished. Remember that recovery is about evolving. Grief is about embracing the loss and entrusting it to a new future. With so many losses, it may feel like a stripping of sorts. You are stripped of your old life and all that it was. And as hard as that is, there is also space to recreate and rebuild at your own pace. No rush. If we believe that God holds all time in His hand (Psalm 31:15a), then we also must watch for His direction – be it closed doors or open windows or different roads altogether. New things are ahead!

You are on track when speaking about grieving who you lost. And believe it or not, grief is a huge marker for recovery because you have the power to remember who you were! But grieving is super-hard. Rest, knowing that you are not alone. God is co-creating with you. What I mean is that you and God can create a new life. With loss there is available space. Ask the Lord to help you build a life that is purposeful. He will help you develop a new life. It takes courage to recognize that you are not the same. It takes perseverance to establish the present self. S/he is evolving too. The brain heals slowly but consistently. Please embrace this new you. Honoring who you were is part of the healing. Embracing the new life is part of the creation. Figuring out your truth is key to building an authentic life. The swirl of loss can be overwhelming. Let your pen and your prayer stabilize you. Journaling offers clarity. Prayer offers comfort. They both offer guidance and healing.

Wondering *why* is natural. Asking *why now* or *why at all* is also natural. Remember that the "why" question tends to be circular, meaning with every answer to why there is another why question. It is better to ask what and how. They offer answers, not more questions. Questioning is part of the anger and bargaining stages of grief. It's OK to ask and to question. God is big enough. Time tends to give us perspective. Pain does too. You may want to check out the book *Prayer in the Night* by Tish Harrison Warren. I hope it will be helpful in some way. One of our brain injury survivors shared that she understood why she survived a horrific car wreck. She recognized that her survival meant that others could live. Years after her wreck, her cousin needed a kidney. She donated one of her kidneys. She also appreciated that her own story of recovery gave other brain injury survivors hope. You will come up with your own reason why. Be patient and watchful. A new understanding will come.

Containment is a helpful exercise when dealing with grief. Colorful boxes and shiny bows are great for gifts, but not for grief and loss. They don't come wrapped beautifully. Like I said, grief is messy. However, you can imagine a precious box (imagine a container with a lid) to secure a memory or person. In your mind's eye, put your memory in the box. It is a sacred space. One that you can grab and ponder, cry over, pray with when you can. And then, place it back for safekeeping. It is always available but not free to roam. After all, we need to function. The precious box gives the memory a container in which to stay while you live your life.

I wanted to talk about "good grief". It is the healthy processing of loss. When one loses oneself to an injury or trauma, especially brain injury, it is extremely difficult to recapture one's previous self. We talked about that a bit earlier. Some have found it helpful to write a goodbye letter to their pre-TBI self and a hello letter to their new self. Grieving is part of the healing process. I have all the hope that you will create the life you want post-TBI. One of our TBI friends painted a rock that symbolized her previous self and painted another rock that symbolized her current self. Find a way to physically demonstrate your experience. It will be a marker from where you can reflect and dream. Some light a candle symbolizing their loss while others create an art piece depicting the person or relationship. You will find your way.

Ambiguous loss…grieving the loss of a person who is physically there but not psychologically/mentally the same person. Ambiguous grief is so tough. One thing that will help you heal through grief is to not force yourself to live in the shadow of someone you are not. There are some attributes that are still part of you. And there are some attributes (personality or experience) that are no longer a part of you. One of our TBI survivor friends said that he likes who he is now more than who he was before the accident. He said that his new self is not so busy and can be more present for his children. I think that practicing gentleness will help you embrace the new you, accept and appreciate the changes. Watch for the parts that are better and more balanced. Continue to extend grace to yourself.

Ambiguous loss…boy, that's a tough one! Mostly because you know it and feel it, yet no one seems to acknowledge it. Many times, loved ones may act like you will forever be impaired instead of changing, growing, and healing. Deficits change, disabilities don't. Honestly, you may be experiencing both deficits and disabilities. That's common. You are in the process of developing new coping strategies. Just remember that grief propels you towards recovery. Even though the grieving (crying, sadness) part of healing feels the worst, it is temporary. Sort of like the last bastion of recovery. The result will feature highlights from your past; appreciation for what/how you survived; and celebration of your new life.

Please consider giving yourself time to grieve and celebrate the lives of those you lost (including your own). Grieve the losses of your former life. There are many. Think about lighting a candle as a testament to the loss of your former self. The lit candle symbolizes a memory, an honoring of someone. This can be a tribute to your former self. As we mentioned, one of the problems with ambiguous loss is the lack of closure. So, think about doing something that marks the end of that person. Watch for your new life to evolve. One day you may feel OK and the next day, not OK. So, extend grace to yourself. You are not alone. With God, every life and loss are redemptive. That's part of His character and His plan. That's what you get to embrace.

Enjoying the new you,
Deana

Homework

- Write a love letter/goodbye letter to the characteristics you miss, to the life that is no longer you. Then write a hello letter to the person you are today.

_____

_____

_____

- Make a list of what you have lost; what you are grieving.

_____

_____

_____

- Make a list of what is being created now.

_____

_____

_____

- Explain what you are discovering about your new self.

_____

_____

_____

Resources

Boss, P. (2010). The trauma and complicated grief of ambiguous loss. *Pastoral Psychology*, 59, 137–145.

Kübler-Ross, E. (1969). *On death and dying*. Charles Scribner's Sons.

Viorst, J. (1986). *Necessary losses*. Simon and Schuster.

Harrison Warren, T. (2021). *Prayer in the night: For those who work or watch or weep*. InterVarsity Press.

Starr, C. (2017). *To root & to rise: Accepting brain injury*. Spiral Path Publishing.

9 Trauma and Stress

I think it's fair to say that experiencing brain injury is both traumatic and stressful. This chapter will delve into both these aspects of brain injury as they relate to the individual and the family. The word "trauma" means wound. The nature of a brain injury is that of a wound to some degree. Whether it is considered mild, moderate, severe, or catastrophic, brain injury is a wound to the brain itself. Stress is defined in several ways, namely emotional or physical strain. Feeling stressed is a normal reaction to challenging experiences such as brain injury. I often say that stress happens when life requires more than our current bandwidth to handle it. Specifically with brain injury, the individual and family are catapulted into a medical world of unknowns. The language is new. The procedures and treatments are new. Typically, there is no previous experience that would give someone the ability to manage such a stressor. So, when you think about it, brain injury can stretch the survivor and family beyond their knowledge or ability to manage it. No matter the degree of the injury, it will stress the individual and family system. As I've often said, when traumatic brain injury (TBI) is diagnosed it is also introduced as the new member of the family, albeit, uninvited. People go into "survival" (do what it takes now to live) mode to get through the crisis. Thankfully, friends and family come alongside to help get through the crisis. They prepare meals, run errands, visit, pray, or bring flowers. However, as we mentioned earlier in the book, support tends to wane (less frequent visits or calls) in part because they think that because the survivor looks normal there is less need for support. The survivor tends to feel alone or like no one cares, which can add to stress because the need for support is still present. The mother of a survivor said that brain injury is a "vulture and life-sucker to so many". Let's break down the two issues.

Trauma

A *traumatic* brain injury indicates that there was some sort of trauma in the experience. The degree of trauma does vary from person to person. If someone experiences a trauma and has symptoms that last more than one month, they are considered to have post-traumatic stress. The symptoms associated with this complicated issue include agitation, anxiety, depression, intrusive thoughts (thoughts that come out of the blue and are hard to get rid of), and nightmares. Sometimes distressing memories, avoidance of anything associated with the traumatic event, feeling detached from loved ones, and feeling numb accompany the emotional struggles. Difficulty having a positive feeling, trouble sleeping, difficulty concentrating or focusing, being easily startled, hypervigilance, and feeling shame and guilt can also be signs of post-traumatic stress. The source of the trauma may be the actual injury experience like in a car wreck or an assault. It can also be medical and treatment experience. For example, some survivors do not remember the actual event but do remember many of the medical tests, X-rays, IVs, etc. Even though it is necessary to survive, hospital experience is an additional source of trauma. If someone has been experiencing any of the symptoms listed at the beginning of the paragraph, my recommendation is to consider working with a licensed mental health professional (licensed professional counselor, social worker, national certified counselor, or psychologist). Ideally, it would be great to work with a counselor/therapist who understands trauma as well as brain injury.

Remember that an event can be traumatic whether you remember it or not. It's hard to say how much someone remembers or does not remember. Sometimes survivors have memory loss of the days before and after the injury. Others experience spotty memories, meaning they remember a snapshot of a scene. For example, Richard, a TBI survivor, remembered that there was a red car but couldn't remember what kind of car it was or why it was on the scene. Research explains that there are times when an accident or event happens so fast that memory is never created. So that means, there is no memory to remember. Most of the survivors that I've worked with say they do not want to remember the accident or whatever caused the brain injury. Patti believes that it is a blessing that she cannot remember. She says that she has no memory of tires squealing or sounds of the crash. She says that she is glad that she does not have those memories to deal with along with everything else.

Trauma Resolution

Trauma resolution, or therapy to help resolve the trauma experienced with brain injury, can be performed through counseling techniques. Basically, counselors can help you work through or process aspects of the experience that are hard to deal with. For those of you who want to talk to a counselor about the traumatic event, you may ask about the following techniques. Eye movement desensitization and processing (EMDR), cognitive-behavioral therapy (CBT), and cognitive processing therapy (CPT) are effective in treating post-traumatic stress disorder (PTSD). I'll explain each of these briefly. In eye movement desensitization and processing (EMDR) a counselor asks you to remember the traumatic event while the counselor moves a visual stimulus such as a pencil or pen from side to side. You do not share the details with the counselor but tell them how it makes you feel. For example, on a scale of 1–10 (high intensity), what number best describes how you feel when thinking about the event? During the therapy, the emotions about the event should feel less intense. The goal is to reduce the emotional charge of the memory.

Cognitive-behavioral therapy (CBT) focuses on changing negative thoughts that make you feel bad. It identifies various wrong or negative thoughts such as all-or-nothing thinking or overgeneralization. Other cognitive distortions are discounting the positive, catastrophizing, and personalization. I'll explain these. All-or-nothing thinking is seeing things as good or bad, black or white. For example, if you make one mistake at work, you think that you are a careless employee. A more realistic thought would be, "I made a mistake. Probably need more training." Overgeneralization uses words like never, always, everything, or nothing. For instance, if a friend misses your call, you may think he never answers his phone when you call. A more reasonable thought would be, "My friend missed my call. She must be busy." CBT identifies several other patterns of wrong thinking and helps the person replace it with more accurate perceptions and beliefs. Discounting the positive is a common faulty thinking pattern with TBI. The survivor tends to discount the positives in his recovery because he is comparing his post-injury self to his pre-injury self. For example, the survivor finally doesn't need a walker, yet he feels bad because he never used one before the injury. Comparing your current self to the non-injured self is an unfair comparison. Because the truth is, you have really done well in being able to walk again! Catastrophizing is when someone believes the worst possible outcome will happen before the event occurs. It is a worst-case-scenario mindset. I think that many people think in this way to survive. What I mean is that sometimes it is safer to predict and prepare for a bad result than to hope for a positive one. An example is when you think that just because you failed a test at school, you will never be able to succeed in life. An alternative way of thinking is if you failed a test, you just failed a test. It has nothing to do with your future. Another common distortion with TBI is personalization. This happens when the person believes that every negative event is somehow his fault. Again, this can be a survival mechanism in that if he believes something is his fault, then he has the power to change the negative outcome in the future. It is best to fight that urge to take things personally. Most of the time, an event or comment has nothing to do with you. Just because your husband is in a bad mood does not mean that you did something wrong. It could be a variety of other issues. The same is true for brain injury. If the survivor is agitated, it does not mean that you said something or did something wrong. It might be because he is tired or hungry or reacting to too much noise. Research says that 95% of rejection has nothing to do with the person. So do your best not to take things personally. Any of these cognitive distortions can have a negative impact on us. It is good to recognize what they are and adjust the way you think towards more reasonable and positive outcomes.

Cognitive processing therapy (CPT) specifically addresses the actual traumatic event and helps the survivor change unhelpful or inaccurate perceptions (ways of thinking). It is more structured because it has a series of strategy worksheets and homework assignments. One homework assignment is to write a detailed account of a traumatic event. Another assignment is to write how the event impacted you and your belief about the world. A strategy that a counselor may use is to help the survivor address stuck points. A stuck point is when you can't move beyond a specific thought or memory. Sometimes it is a question like, "Why did that happen to me?" Sometimes it is when you believe that the incident is all your fault. The goal is to help you rebuild your sense of self and learn more effective coping strategies to deal with the traumatic event. CPT helps you understand what trauma is and how to challenge untrue thoughts about the trauma, such as, "It was all my fault." This technique helps you change unhelpful beliefs to more accurate understanding. Any of these three counseling techniques may be helpful.

Stress

Stress is a normal reaction to daily difficulties. Your body will tell you when you are stressed by a faster heartbeat, sweating, dilated pupils, or hypersensitivity to lights and sounds. There is a positive form of stress otherwise known as good stress or eustress (/ⓧyoōⓧstres/). An example would be when you are discharged from the hospital. It is a good thing but stressful transitioning to home. Bad stress is called distress. When people talk about being stressed out, that is normally what they mean. Having poor stress tolerance (it doesn't take much to make you feel stressed) can be an outcome of brain injury. One survivor told me in one of our sessions, "It's like my stress button is broken. I get stressed super-easy over the smallest things." It is hard to manage stressful situations. Sometimes that is because it is hard to identify what causes stress or if you feel stressed at all. Things that contribute to increased stress are trying to control the uncontrollable (e.g., we can't control what other people do or think), pushing yourself beyond your limits (e.g., making yourself stay up and talk when you really need to rest), dealing with unfair expectations from yourself or others (e.g., "It's been three months since my injury, I should be able to go back to work"), and not being able to say "no" and set healthy boundaries (e.g., letting someone who stays too long visit anyway). Symptoms of stress include fatigue, nausea, anxiety, insomnia, headaches, anger outbursts, restlessness, muscle tension, pain, upset stomach, rashes such as hives, or feeling overwhelmed. Generally, education about brain injury and its impact on the family goes a long way in helping mitigate stress. If the survivor or family member knows what to expect, they can create a game plan to navigate it.

Like stress felt by the survivor, the family also has stressful feelings. The eustress of a loved one coming home from the hospital is both wonderful and stressful. It is good that he is well enough to come home, yet stressful because it will require changes in the environment such as having a bedside commode. Distress or bad stress felt by the family includes financial stress. How will they pay the bills? Often caregivers must take leave from work or change to a part-time schedule. Families feel stress when their loved one recovers slowly. They experience stress when there is limited support from the community and friends. My experience is that caregivers feel significant stress because they feel like they are ill-equipped to manage the recovery of their loved one. Many will tell me that they needed education classes to take so they could understand and prepare for taking care of their loved one. Ashley, the wife of Tim, said, "Why don't these hospitals offer training classes for us like they do for new parents?" Good question.

Handling Stress

So, how can you handle stress as a brain injury survivor or as a caregiver? Consider these strategies and see which ones best fit you and your lifestyle.

1. Practice relaxation techniques. This can be tightening and relaxing each muscle group. Another technique is listening to a relaxation tape such as floating on a cloud (see appendix A). Tai chi and yoga are also great for relaxation. Consider uploading a couple of apps: the Calm app and the Headspace app.
2. Deep breathing. Regulating your breathing helps calm the body and reduce its reaction to stress. Box or square breathing was mentioned in chapter 4.
3. Exercise. Consider walking or practicing gentle movement as a part of your everyday routine. This helps reduce symptoms of stress and increase the ability to manage stress.
4. Write in a journal. Some prefer to journal verbally as in a voice recorder.
5. Eat a healthy diet and avoid a lot of caffeine. Too much carbohydrates, sugar, and caffeine can increase inflammation and reduce the body's ability to manage stress.
6. Spend time on your hobbies. Not only is this productive, it helps you focus on something other than what is stressful.
7. Talk to a friend who gets it. Finding someone who understands brain injury and is willing to talk about it is a rare and beautiful find.
8. Recharge. Do something that makes you feel better.
   a Spend time in nature.
   b Light scented candles.
   c Savor a cup of tea.
   d Play with a pet.
   e Listen to music.
   f Watch a comedy.
   g Curl up with a good book.
9. Practice gratitude. Keep a positive attitude. A predictor for good recovery is keeping a positive outlook. Finding the positive in a difficult situation helps balance the negative and gives hope for the future.
10. Learn to say "no". This is a tough one! As you practice "no", you will find more space in your life to do what you want and need. Here are a few "no" statements:
    a "I wish I could, but I can't right now."
    b "Not at this time."
    c "My schedule does not allow for that."
    d "I do not have the capacity or energy right now."

11 Organize your time.
   a Make a list.
   b Prioritize.
   c Schedule time to accomplish a task.
   d Cross it off when finished.

12 Try not to be hard on yourself. You are doing the best that you can with the resources available to you.

As you manage the stress, think about making a list of triggers. Sometimes you can recognize what causes stress. For example, if someone changes the time of your appointment, it can be more stressful than someone changing the menu. Think of a balloon that is getting overfilled with air; eventually it will burst. Come up with things that stretch you and make you tense. These are probably triggers of stress. Now, let's go to the counseling room and talk more.

Letter to You

Dear Friend,

Trauma and stress can complicate recovery. They can contribute to a slow recovery process mostly because instead of concentrating on the therapies needed to recover, you have to deal with the stress of the environment. For example, you are ready to go to physical therapy, but your ride is late. So, you must change your plans just to get to the therapy. I know you have had similar experiences. That is why we want to get a handle on how to manage them! Sometimes those two issues make you feel different, like you do not recognize yourself. In the case of TBI, stress and trauma tend to be two sides of the same coin. In other words, trauma is on one side of the coin and stress on the other side of the coin. The coin is brain injury. Honestly, I think this is why recovery is so challenging. Sometimes it causes you to feel like you are on the outside looking into your own life. I think this contributes to you feeling alone as well. A fellow survivor wrote a great piece called "Outside, Inside" that I think you will relate to (see Appendix B). As you recover, you will be able to identify stress when it comes. You will get to the place where you usually know what will stress you and what will not. This helps you plan activities that cost the least emotionally. Normally that means doing something that is low key like having coffee with a loved one or listening to your favorite music. Pat, a TBI survivor, said that she sits outside in the sun until she starts to get hot. Also, when your body starts to react with migraines or some other physical symptoms, take a minute and breathe. Scan your stress level or stressors by asking yourself, "Do I feel mild stress or major stress?" Sometimes just recognizing that you and your body are feeling tense, means that it is time to step away from an activity. You may also remind yourself of what is true in that minute. You may say, "I am safe and loved." Remembering what is true helps reduce your stress. Concentrating on what is happening in the minute keeps you from worrying about things in the future.

There is a spiritual component I want to mention. Brain injury recovery can make you feel either closer to or more distant from God, your Higher Power. Please remember that feeling disconnected from God is part of stress, not an indication of your personal relationship. He is always with you whether you feel Him or not. There is so much demanding your attention cognitively, emotionally, physically. Something that I hold on to is that even when the brain or body is hurt, the spirit is intact. In other words, the spirit does not have a TBI. The spiritual part of you holds a separate place. For the Christian faith, this is where we depend on the intercession of the Holy Spirit who prays for us. The Jewish prayer *tikkun olam* means repairing the world. In our day, it includes acts of kindness and charitable giving. Your devotion to recovery and finding your best self encompasses this. Giving to others and telling your story are examples of *tikkun olam*. You can repair people in your world by sharing your recovery with them. Remember you are this world's best-kept secret to resilience. In other words, you have learned so much about living successfully, and we (the world) need to hear it. Tell us your secret to surviving. That is living *tikkun olam*.

Creating sacred space (a place where you and your God meet) involves stillness (holy), quiet, communication with God. He will direct your path. He will be your safe place, your shelter. In those moments, He will also tell you where to go or when to sit in His presence. Our job is to listen and receive. I think you'll find more joy once you've cultivated sacred space. Your specific faith will guide you in how to do this routinely. Whether that is in reciting a homily or prayers or praying the rosary, you will find your specific sacred space. Remember that spiritual practices help reduce stress by increasing good chemicals (neurotransmitters) like serotonin, dopamine, and endorphins. They help improve your mood and can contribute to feelings of happiness and motivation. Ancient religions practiced sacred space while walking labyrinths (a path that symbolizes the ebb and flow of life). They used the etched-out path to help them pray and meditate. You may not have a labyrinth, per se, but you can create a familiar pathway. These pathways or labyrinths are meant to give direction, to symbolize life's journey. Perhaps you can create a labyrinth symbolizing your TBI journey. Consider creating stations that call for you to reflect on certain aspects of your journey. Janice, a TBI survivor, was asked to create a prayer garden at her church. She mapped out a path that had different stopping places. Each stopping place had an activity such as, "Write down three lessons you learned from a stressful experience." The garden had soft music playing in the background so that whoever walked the path also had soft music to listen to. Another one of her stops had paints and rocks. She instructed the person to paint something hopeful on the rock. Labyrinths are meant to create a meditative experience. It is OK to not have directions, though. You're still in God's ICU (He sees you!), meaning you are still in recovery. Allow yourself to dream about what you want your life to look like; about who you want to be. Create a cycle of work, rest, and reflect. Create a routine that is productive for you. Then think about how well it works. Take time to rest. You'll find yourself moving forward with less struggle and more peace.

Reducing the feeling of being overwhelmed is about offloading stress where you can. Offloading can be about delegating, or postponing to a more appropriate time when you have the energy and your cognition is more on point (probably in the mornings). For example, ask for help. Be OK with moving a task to a better time when you can think clearer and have more energy. I like to call it "Operation Energy Conservation". Your health is the priority. Accommodating brain injury is primary. From that, all other responsibilities fall into place. For example, one of my clients was overwhelmed at the holiday stress. She decided to email her well-wishes to family instead of writing cards and going to the post office to mail them. She also decided to minimize decorations. She said that this helps her not feel overwhelmed with time constraints and organizing. Another option for delegating is to ask a friend to run an errand for you. Instead of you going to the store to pick up a few items, your friend can go get what you need. While the family is typically the main caregiver for the survivor, it is wise and helpful to allow friends and community to offer additional support. For example, a church group making meals for a season of time or giving gift cards to various restaurants or stores.

Regarding holidays, let me share a few thoughts on how to manage stress. (For a full discussion, read chapter 11, "Events and Holidays".) These are actually good options for any high-stress event or get-together.

1   Separate when you can to a quiet space or room. Go outside and sit in the sun, if the weather permits.

2   Play calming music or listen to a favorite podcast.
3   Pray.
4   Enjoy nature by looking out of a window or walking slowly outside.
5   Remember to write down the wins in your recovery.
6   Schedule rest according to the event. For example, for every two-hour event, schedule one day or half a day of rest (maybe use a 1:3 ratio: rest three hours/days for every one hour of an event).
7   Manage what you can; release what you cannot. In other words, do not stress over things that are beyond your control. Use your energy to focus on what you can handle.

Two more thoughts to consider about safe space. In your own home, create a peaceful and safe space. Maybe that is a corner of a room or a whole room. Decorate it with things that calm you and give you peace. Let it be a space that allows you to breathe and not worry. The second is to enjoy nature. May I ask you to please take time to walk outside… in between the feelings of being exhausted is a fresh perspective. Think of an Oreo cookie. The top and bottom are "exhausted" and the middle is "perspective". Sometimes taking time to rest and reflect helps us think about things differently. It gives us a fresh perspective. Nature is the best way I know to experience that. So, I'll add another word to your new life…"savor". Move slowly enough to appreciate the experience. Kind of like savoring chocolate. Enjoy the sweetness and depth of flavor of the experience.

Managing triggers is part of managing stress. Triggers are wonderful, painful opportunities to do things differently. It calls for a pivot…to do things differently even if you're not sure what to do. Susan gives us a good example of this. As a grandmother, she loves having her grandchildren in her home. But as a TBI survivor, the noise and chaos that are normal with toddlers trigger a stress response. She and her son worked on a "pivot" which was to only have one toddler at a time for one hour. This offered Susan the opportunity to enjoy her family without experiencing a stressful reaction. I think that you are the best resource for your own healing because internally you know what you need. Most of the time, it is safety and comfort. When you are triggered, please practice peace in the pivot, not panic. For example, reminding yourself that God holds all time in His hands (Psalm 31:15), even the difficult times. Walk away or change the subject when someone triggers you. Recognizing your triggers is a good thing. I do think that feeling exhausted and fatigued is a trigger too. It's like when an infant is too tired to play or do anything except cry. The best way to handle fatigue is rest. Please consider your recovery time with your spouse or partner as a holy respite. Even though it will require energy, it can be a precious time of being together. Ground yourself in what is true right now. Practicing mindfulness is super-helpful in managing stress. Grounding yourself is focusing on all your senses. What are you seeing? What are you hearing? What is the fabric of your shirt? Mindfulness is similar in that you are aware of your thoughts, emotions, and experience in the present moment. Angel, the wife of a TBI survivor, would count ceiling tiles when she was stressed. She said that it helped her focus and calm down.

The anticipation that something bad is going to happen or may happen is a trauma response. This is sort of your brain's way of making you create a safety plan. The problem is, most of the time the thing you worry about happening doesn't ever happen. So, you worry unnecessarily. This is when it might be helpful to create a mantra (a short phrase that you can repeat to yourself). Think of the American folktale "The Little Engine that Could". The little engine did not think he could go up a steep hill. Despite the steep climb and huge load, he was able to slowly succeed by repeating, "I think I can. I think I can." Alli, a TBI survivor, would say to herself, "God's got this" as a way of calming herself during a stressful time. Other mantras shared with me from survivors are, "I am safe." "The Lord is my strength." "I am calm." Anyway, you get the idea. Something that you can say to yourself that automatically grounds you.

Thank you for sharing the deep pain and experiences with me. I count it as an honor. I do believe that you are getting healthier. Hopefully, you are beginning to practice some strategies to help you navigate and resolve past traumas. However painful it feels is the extent of joy to come! Meaning, the depth of pain is the depth of joy. Honor the pain; it tells a story. Celebrate the victory; it gives us hope. Enjoy the small wins; it encourages us to keep trying.

Remember, you are on the road of healing! It's OK to feel all the emotions…anger, sad, ambiguous loss (loss of routine, past life, etc.), regret, etc. That's part of giving yourself a voice to share your story and for acknowledging what you have survived. The other side of grief is noticing and appreciating the bits of joy along the way and maybe even happy moments. Grieving tends to help us focus on what we do have, the joys of what we can do, and the relationships we do enjoy. Keep your eyes open to the bubbles of joy that will peek around the corner when you least expect it.

Watching for joy with you,
Deana

Homework

- Please grab a cool journal and start writing about your FIRSTS (capitalize the letters of first)...there will be many to come! For example, remembering to take your medication without a reminder for the FIRST time. Or brushing your hair without assistance for the FIRST time.
- This one might be a bit challenging... Use the word trauma and create an acrostic for how you manage it. For example, T stands for talk. You can talk to someone you trust about how you are feeling.

T:_____

R:_____

A:_____

U:_____

M:_____

A:_____

- Now create an acrostic for stress. How do you manage stress? For example, S stands for silence. Being quiet helps me feel less stressed.

S:_____

T:_____

R:_____

E:_____

S:_____

S:_____

Resources

Lefaivre, C. (2014). *Traumatic brain injury rehabilitation: The Lefaivre Rainbow Effect.* CRC Press.

Edward, L., & Khan, A. (2019). *Concussion, traumatic brain injury, mTBI ultimate rehabilitation guide: Your holistic manual for traumatic brain injury rehabilitation and care.* Amazon Digital Services LLC.

10 Fatigue and Rest

Fatigue

Fatigue is one of the most common experiences of people who have traumatic brain injury (TBI). It takes the form of mental, physical, cognitive, and emotional fatigue. It's not the same as what most normal people feel. It is not a tired, sleepy feeling. No, for brain injury, fatigue is an all-encompassing unable-to-function event. Yet, some survivors still have to go on and do life. Several survivors through the years have described fatigue in various ways. One friend said that it "feels like walking through cooked oatmeal". Another said that fatigue "feels like I'm cycling into an invisible wind".

It is hard to know why fatigue is so common after brain injury. Typically, it comes more quickly and frequently than among the normal population. Perhaps it is part of the healing process. As the brain heals, it requires more sleep. Think of an infant. The baby sleeps a lot as it grows. It could be because the brain is not working as efficiently. Another reason is that it takes more time, energy, and effort to complete simple tasks. Think about a time when you were exhausted. As a normal person, it was hard for your brain to engage and for you to make decisions. This experience is a fraction of what brain injury folks feel. Add to that the second-guessing they do because they do not have trust in their own brain. This is why the time to complete tasks is extended. One survivor said that everything takes more time and, "I have to think about every step of a task or chore. I can no longer assume I will know what to do without thinking about it." Sleep disturbance contributes to fatigue. Often a TBI survivor may get six to eight hours of sleep but because there is a brain injury, the person may not wake up full of energy. In fact, some survivors say that they wake up at 80% energy. And once they have prepared for their day, most of their energy is depleted. So that while a normal

DOI: 10.4324/9781003602774-10

person's end of workday is at 5pm, a TBI survivor's end of workday may actually need to come at 12 noon.

I've often thought as I've worked with TBI survivors through the years that if they can control their fatigue, they can more easily manage their deficits. So how does one manage fatigue? First, it is important to understand what causes fatigue. Often it is because of sensory overload. Meaning there is too much going on in the environment, such as loud noises, bright lights, uncomfortable temperatures, or too many people. That overload can be visual, auditory, emotional, or physical. We will talk about each of these below. Fatigue can sometimes be caused by too much pain. Whatever the trigger (and it could be different every time), it is important for the survivor and his care partner to understand the cause to help manage or avoid it. Lastly, low barometric pressure can cause fatigue and other issues because of the swelling of blood vessels and tissues around the brain. Other issues are headaches, brain fog, dizziness, joint pain, balance struggles, and lack of alertness. As much as possible, removing yourself from the triggers is best. Sometimes that means resting. Or, if that is not possible, retreat to a quiet location. Rachel, a TBI survivor, would go to her car and rest when she was overwhelmed at a restaurant. She would be quiet and rest her eyes and then she was ready to go back to the restaurant.

Auditory Overload

Auditory overload contributes to fatigue. It can come in the form of noises that are too loud. Or sometimes it is a slight agitation that magnifies for the survivor such as someone tapping his pencil or shifting in his seat or an unbalanced ceiling fan. Auditory overload also occurs when there is too much cross talk. Most social and family events with more than a couple of people involve more than one person speaking at the same time. Once when I was working in the emergency department of a local hospital, a patient came in with a TBI. His family members were piled into the same little room trying to talk to him. He became more and more agitated and unable to carry on with a conversation. The family was asked to appoint one family member to attend to him. After they left and he was able to rest, he became less agitated, less confused, and more responsive. Removing the auditory overload and giving him a moment to rest was what he needed to continue working with the treatment team. Other sources of auditory overload include radio, music, and television sounds. Environmental sounds can contribute to auditory overload.

Sounds such as a leaky faucet, background music, white noise machine, or distant traffic such as honking cars, trains passing, or airplane traffic. Remember to use earplugs, sunglasses, or a hat to help reduce stimulation. Sometimes, just walking away and being alone is all that is needed. You will know what is best for you.

Visual Overload

Anything within one's field of vision can cause visual overload. From bright lights to movies to reading can independently cause fatigue for a survivor. In my practice, I am aware of the sensitivity of individuals to lights. So, to alleviate some of the visual stress, I have low-intensity lighting. Sometimes I must turn those off as well. One client with TBI could only manage ambient lighting from the hall. She could not sit facing a window because of the visual distractions. Sometimes wearing sunglasses can help the survivor manage the light intensities. Riding in a car can be particularly difficult. Not only watching traffic and passing images, but the speed of the car can also contribute to visual overload. Some survivors have difficulty processing speed as well as perceiving two- or three-dimensional objects. Also, keeping an orderly environment is helpful for survivors. Simple decorations or accessories are easier to process. Plus, if possible, keep things the same. Changing décor or furniture creates difficulty for the survivor because it is unfamiliar and will require additional processing. Clutter is to be minimized to avoid visual overload. A speech therapist shared a coping strategy for visual overload. She said to close your eyes for a few seconds (if you can do so without getting dizzy). When we close our eyes, it automatically preserves 40% of the brain's energy. Applying light, gentle pressure or a warm washcloth over your eyes can help clear the vision. It creates a "reset" of one's vision.

Physical Overload

Helping the survivor focus on one thing at a time can help avoid physical overload. Stamina and endurance are built over time. It is important to recognize the physical limitations of the survivor and encourage staying within suggested guidelines of movement. Some rehabilitation centers and outpatient therapies utilize yoga (specific to brain injury) to help improve endurance, stamina, and flexibility for the survivors. Remember that exercise can be simply movement. It does not always mean a formal workout, especially at the beginning of recovery. It can mean walking, doing chair exercises, or stretching. Be aware of the outside elements such as humidity, temperature, and wind speed, all of which contribute to physical exertion and possible overload. These elements contribute to the difficulties with barometric pressure changes. Additionally, the level of pain can cause physical overload. Sometimes it is difficult to ascertain what is causing the pain. The survivor and care partner may want to investigate the pain with their primary physician. One of the most common pain problems are headaches and, sometimes, migraines. Some survivors also complain about nerve pain. Either one of these sources can be helped with the assistance of a pain management physician.

Emotional Overload

Any type of stress can contribute to emotional overload for a survivor. Stress management is recommended for family members as well as the survivor. Techniques include activities that take your mind off stressful situations. For example, do something that is creative, whether it is coloring or building something or polishing jewelry. Physical movement such as walking gives an outlet for stressful feelings. Practicing relaxation techniques like deep breathing or visualization meditation is helpful to reduce stress. Visiting with friends can be a natural way of getting your mind off the stress and onto the conversation. Sometimes it just takes a break to get you through a stressful time. The changes in roles, expectations, abilities, dreams, and financial resources all contribute to stress within the home. Some of these role changes include using energy for therapies instead of doing household chores. Relationship changes are when the survivor needs more care and therefore more supervision. In those moments, the survivor is not able to perform as the partner he was before. Sometimes changes in abilities create stress, especially when you can remember what you could do before the injury. And as with any catastrophic illness, financial resources are depleted, which becomes a major stressor for the family. Remember that survivors often have lost the "filter" that can sift out unwanted stress. They can feel or pick up on the vibe of a room or a feeling from a loved one. Because there is more exposure, there is also a tendency to feel uncomfortable and overloaded emotionally.

Energy Conservation

Fatigue demands that we conserve as much energy as possible. Scheduling activities according to how much energy they will cost is vital. So, for example, a TBI survivor who is early in his recovery may only plan one big event per week. Then, plan to rest for up to three days afterwards because the brain is trying to repair, and your body is trying to re-live. It takes loads of energy. Especially in the early stages of recovery, a major event may be simply showering. If that is all that can be accomplished that day, and you do accomplish it, then it is a good day. As recovery continues, one task can grow into two or more tasks per day. Again, consider the completion of those tasks as successful steps in recovery. Congratulate yourself for doing that one big thing and for doing the small things. I want you to be your own cheerleader as you learn to live again. It is important to remember that recovery from TBI is inconsistent. So that means, even if one feels well enough to accomplish three tasks in one day, it may still be the case that one cannot function at that same level the next day. Let your brain and body tell you the right pace and rhythm for doing activities. As we've talked about previously, the most consistent thing about TBI is that it is inconsistent. This is one of the reasons survivors and family members have difficulty understanding the projected recovery. What I tell my clients is to look at the "30,000-foot view" as well as the "10-foot view" of recovery. In other words, try to see the progress from a large picture view and a small picture view. The greater the perspective, the more one will realize the progress. It is not a day-to-day progression but rather a month-to-month progression. As a counselor, typically progress is not evident from session to session, but it can be identified after several sessions. This is another reason why it is important to compare your current self with the self who was first injured. You will see huge recovery steps even when you may not have noticed them day-to-day. Journaling can also help document recovery. Our TBI survivor, Patti, would write in her journal every "First" since her wreck. After several years of recovery, she is still able to write "Firsts" in her life after brain injury. The same can be true for every survivor.

Signals of Fatigue

Every survivor is different in how they experience fatigue. However, there are common symptoms that signal to the survivor that he needs to slow down and rest. Here are a few ways one can experience fatigue:

- Feeling cold.
- Being irritable.
- Experiencing brain fog.
- Becoming pale.

- Trying to push through fatigue to complete a task.
- Nausea.
- Loss of control of emotions.
- Blurry vision.
- More talkative.
- Easily distracted.
- Restless.
- Glazed expression.
- Tense look.
- Denial of feeling fatigued.
- Dizziness.
- Inability to concentrate or focus.
- Difficulty being redirected.
- Rubbing your face or forehead.
- Not giving as much eye contact.

Perhaps you have experienced some of these symptoms. And you may have your own signals that you are fatigued. Patti, our TBI survivor, says that when she is fatigued, "my 'irritability thermometer' raises in no time at all. Fatigue zaps and steals my energy." The bottom line is: listen to your body and your brain. They will not lead you wrong but rather give you direction on how to manage fatigue.

Managing Fatigue

We talked earlier about certain practices that will help one manage fatigue. I believe it is helpful to narrow it down to four categories: pacing, prioritizing, sleep hygiene, and exercise. Pacing is vital to create a productive day. Years ago, I came up with a saying, "Add grace to your pace." In other words, do not push yourself to accomplish more than your body and brain can handle. One of the reasons that people become fatigued is that they try to push themselves past what they have the bandwidth for. In other words, a situation requires more than they can do. I've noticed through the years that people who consider themselves to have a "type A" personality tend to want to heal with the same kind of gusto. Being a high performer, fast mover, or a quick thinker may have been a part of your personality. However, with brain injury, the same enthusiasm has a greater impact on your fatigue levels. And that's OK. It is OK to give yourself a break and not push so hard. And it is just as important for the caregivers to allow for mistakes and slower pacing. Try not to expect the survivor to behave or perform as he did prior to the injury. That is where grace comes in. Extending grace is like being kind to yourself or your loved one and understanding the limitations. It is about being courteous and thoughtful to oneself during a challenging day. Pushing yourself beyond your current ability is mean. It is the same as making someone drive 100 miles when they only have 25 miles' worth of gasoline. Pushing beyond the limits guarantees more mistakes and possible setbacks in recovery. So, be kind and gracious to yourself. You are doing the best that you can.

Another part of pacing is scheduling the cognitively hard tasks during the time of day when you are most alert. Also, scheduling one major task per day can be helpful in managing fatigue. Of course, every survivor is different. And as one recovers, the ability to accomplish more than one or two tasks per day will increase. One survivor reported that she tries to do three things each day: one physical task such as walking; one cognitive task such as pouring her medication; and one spiritual task such as praying or meditating. Another pacing exercise is scheduling rest periods. That may mean simply closing your eyes for a few minutes. Sometimes it may mean taking a short nap. Whatever the case, resting is very important in successful brain injury recovery. If you have traveled in traffic to an appointment, chances are that the drive has fatigued you. In those cases, pacing means allowing for an extra 30 minutes to 1 hour to simply relax. Several of my TBI survivor clients schedule time to rest before the session and time to rest after the session and before they get back on the road to drive home. They give themselves mental and physical cushions on each side of an appointment. Pacing can include what I call taking a "therapeutic break" from all the appointments. Especially early on in the recovery process, survivors are required to attend several therapy or doctor appointments each week. They tell me that they are fatigued from going to all the appointments. In those cases, it can be helpful to take a week off from all the activities to rest and recuperate. Taking a therapeutic break can give the survivor an opportunity to refocus and reset.

Prioritizing is a great coping strategy that helps manage fatigue. As I mentioned earlier, sometimes the morning is the best time to complete harder cognitive tasks. One may consider scheduling therapy or other appointments earlier in the day as a means for lessening fatigue. The main reason for prioritizing is planning each activity according to one's capability. Prioritizing also means letting go of activities that you no longer enjoy. It may be helpful to ask someone to come alongside of you to help with the task. After brain injury, some survivors have different likes and dislikes. What once was enjoyable (such as snowboarding or sailing) is no longer enjoyable. Give yourself space to learn the new you. Prioritizing the enjoyable activities can go a long way in helping you appreciate how you have changed. Writing lists helps you to organize and prioritize. Some survivors use their electronic device to keep notes and lists. Others use sticky notes and place them in high-traffic areas in their home. Lists and notes help relieve fatigue. One of the survivors stated that he keeps his notes on his phone and refers to them as often as necessary. He also takes a picture of what he wants to remember such as a parking space.

It stands to reason that sleep hygiene will contribute to reducing fatigue. Sleep is necessary to function and to recover. The difficulty is that most people do not have a good understanding of how to practice good sleep hygiene. Let me give you a few suggestions. Create the same sleep routine each night. For example, set a bedtime that is consistent each day. Preparing for bed normally includes brushing your teeth, taking a bath or shower, or meditating and praying. Whatever you do to prepare for bed, continue the same routine. This signals to your body and brain that you are in the process of going to sleep. Some things to avoid are drinking caffeine, watching stimulating television or movies, and being on your electronic device. Avoiding screen time helps reduce the exposure of blue light which inhibits the release of melatonin. Blue lights trick your brain into thinking it is daytime. Winding down before bed may include reading or coloring or stretching. The goal is to do something relaxing. Preparing your bedroom to be conducive to sleep means tidying up and eliminating clutter; avoiding noises and lights; cooling the temperature; and turning down the bed.

Exercising during the day can help the body prepare to sleep at night. Exercising safely is very important in recovery to help the body become stronger and to prepare for sleep when it is time. It is not suggested to do strenuous exercise at night. However, low-impact exercise such as yoga can help the body relax. Think of exercise as movement. This will help you not feel overwhelmed when thinking of a one-hour workout. Movement in walking a few extra steps per day. Or doing additional household chores. Exercise helps us feel more positive and improves energy levels. It provides a host of health benefits such as strengthening heart function, building bone density, improving muscle tone, lowering stress, reducing risk of osteoporosis, and managing weight.

Often, fatigue and rest go together. When you are fatigued, rest becomes the first plan of attack so to speak. It is important to remember that rest is not about being lazy but about allowing your brain and body to reset for more activity. You may notice that as recovery continues, fatigue is less of an issue. In other words, you may not need as much rest because you are able to function for an extended amount of time. It is important to identify what triggers fatigue for the survivor. Is it a specific task? Is fatigue more evident during the rainy season? Does being around a lot of people contribute to fatigue? Does listening to someone talk trigger fatigue? There may be a myriad of reasons that cause fatigue, from a specific task, to the environment, expectations, an external stimulus, or getting sick. It is helpful to recognize what specifically causes fatigue and then create game plans to rest and recover. Now, let's talk about it in the counseling room.

Letter to You

Dear Friend,

Fatigue...this is a huge one! Please listen to your body and brain. If you need to rest, rest. If you can't take a nap, close your eyes. That preserves 40% of your brain's energy. At any rate, this is not the time to push yourself. It's not nice. And you deserve to be treated nicely! Remember, your fatigue calls the shots. If you're done, be done. It will serve you better in the long run if you listen and pay attention to fatigue. If you can manage your fatigue, you will experience less of the symptoms of TBI. For example, you will feel overwhelmed less quickly and/or become irritated less severely. Do your best not to push yourself...allow for the nap; allow for the body to catch up to the heart; allow for the brain to catch up to the body. Please rest as much as possible. The brain fatigue is one thing...the heart fatigue is something else. Brain fatigue requires unplugging and quiet. It is when you're depleted and cannot do anything more. Heart fatigue (when you feel emotionally exhausted) requires tears, expression, and communion. It means that you need a friend who will listen and not judge, not give an opinion, just be in your presence. Ask the Lord for them.

TBI recovery creates its own timetable. Do your best to honor it instead of pushing. Your processing may take a bit longer. That is about processing, not IQ. When you are cognitively fatigued, it may feel like the brain moves slower. That is OK. Allow for it and be gracious to yourself. Decision-fatigue is fatigue that comes when life requires more than your bandwidth. In other words, you are already at your limit and do not have any energy to decide – even a simple decision like what to eat. People ask you questions or require you to answer or give direction; it amounts to huge cognitive fatigue! What I mean is that simple conversation can put you over the edge because your brain is already tired. Again, giving yourself the space to rest, slow the pace, laugh, smile, or walk will help restore that energy. Your presence is doing your part. Just being there as an observer means a lot to people. Remember that, most likely, you are already considered a hero because of how much you have overcome! No need to add to the conversation when your presence is doing the talking. Let that be enough when the resources are spent. Please do your best to honor yourself and your guests by taking micro-breaks or full rest. We all need it, and I think you're leading the way. Saying, "Please excuse me. I'll rejoin you in one hour," will give them permission to rest too. The speed of the pace only matters if it is too fast. So, be OK with slower pacing.

Look back at the signals that could let you know you are getting fatigued. What signals do you see in yourself? If you experience any of these, add a rest period whether it is ten minutes or two hours. You will find your rhythm (your optimal pace). Do your best not to push yourself, especially when fatigue sets in. Pushing yourself typically leads to more mistakes and exaggerates the deficits you do have. I'm so thankful that you are listening to your body and your brain. This is not the norm with some TBI survivors. They will push themselves too hard and it costs them in the end. When one rests, one multiplies one's time. There is less vacillating with decisions, more clarity, less frustration, more grace. See how adding grace to your pace positively impacts your recovery?

Sleep is another one of those practices that can contribute to reducing brain fog or fatigue, and increasing brain energy. Sticking with a routine around bedtime will help you. Like we talked about, practice sleep hygiene. It is more important than you realize. Most TBI folks wake up with only 50% capacity. Therefore, your 5pm (a normal person's end of the business day) is really 12pm/noon (a survivor's end of the business day). So, if you can schedule hard things in the morning, you will be less likely to feel worn out at the end of the day. Plus, during sleep the glymphatic system is at work. This is a system in the brain that works at night when you are sleeping. It is considered the garbage disposal of the brain because it cleans out old or dead neurons or chemicals that are no longer necessary. Also, TBI fatigue and a normal person's fatigue are completely different. Normal people think that sleep is the ticket for rejuvenation. While that is helpful, it is not the full answer for TBI fatigue. And most TBI people do not get restorative sleep because of the brain injury. They wake up tired instead of refreshed. For TBI, pacing activity, having a quiet environment, adding rest periods, and sleep are all helpful for recovery. As you recover, you will be able to do more, but for now, this "schedule"

122   Fatigue and Rest

will be helpful. As you move into your new normal, one thing to keep in mind is pace. When your deficits (memory, self-anger, etc.) show themselves, let it be a sign for you to step back for a minute and rest. What I mean by rest is doing one of the following:

- Closing your eyes for a few minutes.
- Distracting yourself by changing the subject or doing a different activity.
- Reducing environmental stimulation (lower lights, turn off radio, etc.).
- Slowing down.

Sometimes with a brain injury, your energy wears down like a battery. It's best to pay attention and give yourself mini-breaks along the day. Finding a minute to rest can be difficult when there are responsibilities as a spouse, parent, employee, etc. It is said that President John F. Kennedy would intentionally close his eyes and think about things not office related for a few minutes every hour. It gave him a brief break before attending to his responsibilities.

Let me share with you a few more thoughts. To accommodate flooding (feeling overwhelmed or overloaded) and fatigue… try to schedule one big event per day. For example, one appointment or one thing that will require most of your cognition and brainpower such as a social event. Allow yourself to rest the remainder of the day. Use rest as medicine. Another win is that when you are "done" or have had "enough" you retire to a quiet space. That offers you a place to rest and rejuvenate, reflect and restore. Your family honoring that space is super-important by leaving you alone for a period of time, not creating extra work, not doing just one more thing. The next time you feel like you are doing too much, please stop and take a break. For example, walk away or rest or do something completely different. Then, if you have energy and cognitive bandwidth, go back. Please balance the fatigue with gratitude that you have been able to perform well. Now, rest, please.

Finally, let's talk about meditation. Research has shown that meditation helps manage fatigue and helps you control emotions. It is also helpful to reduce stress and pain. Several religions use meditation as part of their practice and worship. Let me explain a bit about each. Buddhists practice a unique form of meditation called koan, a riddle without an answer. It is meant to demonstrate the inadequacy of reason or logic. Meditation is a core practice of Judaism. Meditation includes ancient texts as well as focus on the symbols of divinity such as Wisdom, Understanding, Knowledge, Mercy, Beauty, Glory, Foundation, and Kingdom. Christianity practices meditation through repeated prayers either individually or corporately. Islam focuses on the teachings of Muhammad in the Koran. Meditation is through spoken words, chant, or song. Muslims also use sacred activities such as dance, writing, calligraphy, and weaving as a means of practicing unity. In Islam, the meditation called *fikr* is meant to prevent the mind from going astray while the heart focuses on God. Lastly, Hinduism uses various spiritual practices including meditation. It plays a part in all areas of spiritual life. One of the main mediations is called dhyana, a yoga practice. It is a means of focusing on the unchanging Lord. Whatever your faith is, lean into the experience.

My hope for you is to realize that fatigue comes with healing. It is not a negative statement about you as a person. It is OK to be fatigued. It is OK to find time to rest, whether it is closing your eyes or meditating. Whatever you choose, it is something that you can practice almost anywhere. And the good news is that rest and meditation are non-pharmaceutical ways of managing fatigue! It is medicine for a tired brain and body.

Add grace to your pace,
Deana

Homework

- List at least three triggers that cause you to feel fatigue.

_____

_____

_____

- List a good schedule for you to rest during each day. What would it look like?

_____

_____

_____

_____

- List four things that help you manage and cope with fatigue.

_____

_____

_____

_____

Resources

McDonald, S., Little, A., & Robinson, G. (2019). *Rebuilding life after brain injury.* Routledge.

Fong, A. (2024). How to overcome neural fatigue from a brain injury. *Cognitivefxusa.* Available at https://www.cognitivefxusa.com/blog/neural-fatigue-after-brain-injury-tbi (accessed November 11, 2024).

Osborn, C. (2000). *Over my head: A doctor's own story of head injury from the inside looking out.* Andrews McMeel Publishing.

11 Events and Holidays

Holidays

As of this writing, the United States is preparing for the holiday season. While it is an exciting time to celebrate various events and holidays, it is also very stressful. Especially stressful when trying to enjoy the holiday with a brain injury because of sensory sensitivities, changes in routine, or high-intensity family experiences. So, I thought it would be helpful to address how to manage events with the least amount of stress. Remember that brain injury survivors tend to become overwhelmed quite easily. More so when there is a change in routine, an increase in activity, and an established deadline to maneuver. When I speak of events, I am referring to celebrations, holidays, shopping trips, medical appointments, extended visits and appointments, sports activities, the arts, moving locations, and memorials. For those without the challenge of brain injury, most holidays and events are demanding physically, emotionally, and mentally. Patti, a TBI survivor, says that some of the issues she has to manage are figuring out if she has enough money, dealing with feelings of putting herself down, attending faith-based programs, and dealing with the grief of not having the same experience as before the brain injury. Preparing for events can be difficult due to the emphasis on executive function such as planning, organizing, and problem-solving. Whether it is a birthday, anniversary, retirement, bar mitzvah, baby shower, festival, or holiday, each requires preparation and planning. Therapy is another event and is not an easy process. It requires a lot of energy and physical and cognitive exertion. Driving to and from the appointment also causes energy depletion. So, please extend kindness to yourself and plan for rest/recovery after each session.

When visiting with friends or family, ask for a room that is relatively quiet where the survivor can retire as needed. Some call it a safe space that is removed from the noise of a gathering. One of our survivor friends shared that he would ask to excuse himself from a conversation, telling the hosts that he will rejoin them in 30 minutes. He then takes his leave and rests in a separate room. Providing a safe space and monitoring fatigue are two coping strategies that will help create a successful visiting experience.

Travel

Another aspect of celebrating or attending events is the travel involved. Whether the travel is by coach, car, train, or plane, it is important to plan for the experience. Planning includes figuring out how many stops there will be, how long there is between stops, how many times luggage is checked, and the type of seating. These extensions in a trip need to be accounted for in order to safely manage the trip. Louise, a TBI survivor, wanted to see her sister in a different state. She knew that flying would not be possible due to the remote location. So, she decided to travel by train. Louise's daughter scheduled the trip so that her mother would not have to change trains during stops. She also planned Louise's snack and packing needs for an extended excursion. Louise was briefed of the stops and what would be required of her. Louise packed sunglasses, earplugs, and a cap to help with possible sensory overload. She was also given two emergency contacts: one with the railroad and one who was a family member. Similar plans can be adapted to coach, car, and plane travel. Having a travel manager can be very helpful for the survivor.

Depending on the severity of the brain injury as well as the location of the injury, travel can vary in the levels of stress it causes. For example, someone injured in a motor vehicle wreck tends to struggle being in a car. The kinesthetic stimuli or sense of movement (vibrations common in vehicles) can cause anxiety and panic. This may be because the body remembers the jolt of a wreck in the past and anticipates it in the present. The reason for the panic sense is that the amygdala (the 24-hour security guard of your brain) is alerted when there is potential harm. The amygdala sets off the fight/flight response which is felt as anxiety and panic. So, it is the brain working on your behalf, not a personal characteristic. Sometimes when someone's vision is involved, watching incoming traffic or noticing passing scenery can contribute to overstimulation. Sometimes survivors experience panic because they see two-dimensionally, not three-dimensionally. Therefore, objects appear closer and faster than they are. Vision problems are not processing the appropriate speed of things or are processing one or two seconds later than the event. Sometimes it is seeing things closer than they are. Vision issues after brain injury contribute to a lot of different reactions when driving or riding. Some survivors have adjusted by focusing on something inside the car instead of watching things out of the window. Others have calming music playing. Still others use medication to help reduce the anxiety of being in a vehicle.

When traveling, be aware of the effects of vibrations (back and forth movement) and frequencies (number of times an object vibrates within a moment of time). Most of the time, the body and brain pick up on the stimuli before the person is aware of it. Typically, it is better to sit at the front of the coach or aircraft. The further in the back you sit, the greater the vibrations that your brain and body must manage. Crowds are another source of stress and sensory overload when traveling. Crowds expose the survivor to cross talk, increased noise, and pressured movement like standing in line when people are too close. I recommend survivors board the aircraft as early as possible to avoid the pressure of finding seats and stowing luggage. Boarding early can also reduce exposure to other passengers. Robert, a TBI survivor, asked his physician to write a note asking for preferred boarding due to his medical condition. This allowed Robert to be seated and ready for the flight before having to deal with other passengers boarding. If possible, have a travel buddy who understands the needs of your brain injury. Travel buddies can locate terminals, restrooms, restaurants, and luggage areas and help navigate the brain injury survivor to the destination needed. A travel buddy is someone aware of your needs as a survivor. He is the designated person dedicated to doing the planning and organizing the trip. He would secure the room closest to the elevator in a hotel, for example. This person can also be assigned to take the survivor to the airport, for example, and retrieve him once he arrives to the destination. Explaining to family or care partners how to help minimize the stress of an airport or coach or train station goes a long way in planning and reducing stress. Essential is communicating clearly so that the survivor and family members understand what is expected.

Another issue to consider in traveling is the terrain and environmental conditions. Terrain changes (grass, asphalt, sand, snow, ice, etc.) can cause frustration or confusion, and make it difficult for the survivor to navigate. Caregivers need to research on how to help their loved one walk and maneuver in unfamiliar places. It is important to plan for external noises and factors such as stairs, uneven pavement, poorly lit passages, wind, rain, snow, heat, and cold weather. The goal is for the survivor to feel comfortable and safe. Also, consider the humidity and barometric pressure, which when high can contribute to brain fog for the survivor. Several years ago, Patti and I were traveling to Vail, Colorado to speak at an international conference. We anticipated some of the details of the trip itself. Precautions were made to accommodate the time, temperature, and terrain changes. We planned frequent stops to rest and booked extended hotel accommodation for one day before the conference and one day after the conference. This allowed for rest and recovery. Pacing was important in that there were so many seminars to attend as well as our own speaking event. Pacing was also needed to allow for needed sleep and rest periods. Other plans were to reserve tables at local restaurants or in the hotel. It is helpful to request tables outside of the high-traffic areas of a restaurant. During our trip we had the opportunity to go to a ski lodge. This meant special care was taken to stay balanced when walking, climbing stairs, and disembarking from a gondola. These newer experiences require a lot of concentration for the survivor, so it is important to keep talking to a minimum. It is helpful to give a short directive to inform the survivor. For example, one could inform the survivor, "The gondola will be approaching in one minute." And then celebrate with the survivor for being able to navigate well!

Hotel accommodation needs may vary with the survivor. Overall, it is recommended to secure a room away from outside noises. Some survivors prefer to stay close to the elevator. Others prefer to stay on the first floor. One of our care partners shared ways that she planned for her daughter, a TBI survivor, to stay at a resort hotel alone. With her daughter's permission, she contacted the hotel concierge and asked him to touch base with her every day. She asked her daughter to also call her each evening. The daughter said that she wanted to spend a few days alone to see if she would be able to take care of herself and have a positive experience. The result of the solo vacation experiment was that the daughter stated that she had felt scared but was glad that she had done it. She was able to take care of herself and enjoy her time at the resort. Her mother stated that she had been anxious and nervous about her daughter being so far away but felt assured because she had at least two contacts each day confirming she was safe. Another family reserved a hotel room for their survivor during a family move, to protect their loved one from the stress of packing and moving. Although it is more expensive to reserve a room, the family believed it to be worth the cost to ensure their loved one would be safe, have meals, and be exposed to less stress.

Events

Worship gatherings can be a struggle for survivors. Examples of worship venues are a mosque, temple, church, shrine, cathedral, gurdwara, synagogue, or chapel. Worship experiences can be challenging due to the crowds, music, choral pieces, or congregational singing. Also, listening to liturgy or messages can be difficult depending on the speaker. If the leader speaks too fast, it will be hard for the survivor to process the information. If the speaker does not speak clearly, it may be difficult for the survivor to hear the consonants in words. Many survivors report having flooding (overloading) experiences because of the lighting, volume of music, cross talk, people, and length of the service. To best serve survivors and others who have sensory challenges, the church may consider having a separate room equipped with a television where they can watch the service. If a separate room is not available, it is recommended for the facility to provide earplugs. To avoid or at least reduce the flooding (being overwhelmed from the various sensory objects), the survivor can wear sunglasses and a hat or cap to reduce the effects of lighting. Concert earplugs seem to be the most helpful for survivors. Sitting close to the exit door can also be helpful to allow the survivor to leave the event safely. Consider seating that is close to doors to allow for easier access for entry and exit. This keeps the survivor from having to navigate large crowds to leave an event. If the survivor is fatigued, it is important he does not push himself beyond what he can safely do. As a caregiver, you may advise your loved one to tell you if he is starting to feel overwhelmed. If so, you can help remove him from the stressors and retreat to a quieter space. Remember that fatigue happens in part because the survivor does not have a filter system in place to filter out external noise, reverberations, lights, etc. Normal people can focus and tune out certain environmental issues. Unfortunately, survivors cannot tune things out, so it makes concentration difficult and the situation overwhelming. Having difficulty in managing distractions seems to be an issue at most stages of recovery.

During sporting events, the above suggestions of wearing earplugs (concert earplugs or ear buds are the most effective at cancelling out noise), sunglasses, and/or a ball cap can reduce environmental sensory stimulation (sounds of the game, noise of the crowd, loud talking, flashing lights, etc.). In addition, one may consider securing seating closer to the aisle for easy access. When navigating steps or an escalator, the care partner may stand in front of the survivor going down and stand behind the survivor when traveling up. This offers extra support should the survivor lose balance. Elayne, a TBI survivor, asks her spouse to hold her hand or allow her to put her hand on his shoulder for stability. It can also buffer the pressure of the crowd. Using handrails is important to maintain stability while navigating stairs or escalators. One of our survivor friends tells her care partner to make sure she can use the handrail on her left side, the stronger side for her.

Other events to prepare for include weddings, parties, graduations, or even grocery shopping. Just a word about grocery shopping. Use a list of items instead of trying to remember what is needed. Also, consider the potential stress of checking out with sounds such as bells, or machines making noises. The stress of exchanging money or using credit cards is an extra pressure that survivors have to navigate. Again, ask a caregiver to help with the shopping. Aubrey, a TBI survivor, asked her husband to check out because she could not handle the stress of standing, waiting, and listening to all of the chimes, bells, cross talk, etc. She said that she was able to locate the items but could not manage the check-out process. She also used the grocery cart to help stabilize her when walking. Similar coping strategies work for these events (weddings, parties, graduations) too. Here is a summary:

- Secure seats close to the exits.
- Pack sunglasses, hats, and earplugs.
- Plan for an early exit when fatigued.
- Ask your spouse or caregiver to assist as needed.

As with any event, it is important to give the survivor space and permission to participate as much or as little as needed. This offers freedom to be present, rest, or be separate depending on the energy and fatigue level of the survivor. And if the survivor says he is too tired to go, believe him. He should have the option to participate or decline even up to the last minute. Let's go to the counseling room and hear a bit from the therapist.

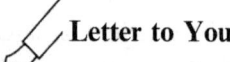

Letter to You

Dear Friend,

The holidays have their own set of challenges! Please pace yourself, especially during the special events. Pacing means not pushing yourself. It means doing one thing, assessing how you feel, and if you feel OK, do the next thing. If you are feeling fatigued or irritable, give yourself permission to stop. The more dissociated you feel, the more you need to rest. That's the brain's way of giving itself space. Please do not push. Pushing yourself is not helpful and unfortunately, it may cost you physically. Please remember to schedule rest (time to be by yourself in quiet or do whatever you need to calm down or put yourself at ease) in all of the holiday events. Extend grace to yourself by allowing for the lower output, meaning if you can only handle a couple of tasks, let that be enough. It's OK. Do your best to let the experience trump (be more important than) the things. Your presence is the greatest gift of all. If you feel like you are about to shut down, take time away for as long as you can and breathe, rest, pet the cats, or do whatever calms you down. The goal is for you to put as much energy into reserve before the holiday and then to plan for recovery afterwards. Recovery means giving yourself a day or two of rest before requiring yourself to do another event. If you've had enough and are "done", please let the family know that you will need to excuse yourself and will join them at a later time. Remember, add grace to your pace.

"Energy conservation" is your mantra for the month! Please consider adjusting expectations to match your capabilities and energy. Sometimes we have time but not energy. Making things simpler can enrich the family experience. There's a Dutch word, *"gezellig"*, which is not translatable in English, but it means: coziness with the loved ones. Consider *gezellig* as your holiday goal instead of the decorations, traditions, etc. Corrie ten Boom was a Dutch watchmaker who was imprisoned in the Holocaust for protecting and saving Jews in Holland during World War II. After the war, she traveled the world sharing about her faith in Jesus and the importance of forgiveness. (For more information, read her biography, *The Hiding Place*.) She had an interesting perspective about things or material possessions. She would often say, "Oh child, it doesn't have eternal life."

Here are a few suggestions for surviving the holiday:

1 Please give yourself permission to take a "break" from all the noise/people/sensory input that comes with the holidays. The rest is for recovery and replenishing.
2 Please allow yourself two to three days after the holiday to recover. Think 3:1 ratio…it takes three days to recover from one day of activity. As your brain heals, kind of watch for how much recovery time you need. Also, drink plenty of water.
3 Give yourself space at any time, and let your family know if you need it. You get a "free pass" to excuse yourself at any time on any day.

4. As much as possible, reduce sensory overload, which means...do not have the TV on when you're trying to talk to one another; try not to talk over one another; and turn on low lights to reduce brightness.
5. Keep visits short with family and friends. You will know how much your brain can handle.
6. When planning for holiday time, remember to factor in the potential travel stress. So, if you have a driving time of two hours, remember that your visit time may need to be shortened to accommodate the extra travel.
7. Also, consider mini-breaks within events such as walking outside or going somewhere quiet. Closing your eyes for a few seconds can also help recharge your energy.
8. Be aware of external noise. If you can, reduce any unnecessary sounds such as music or television or loud talking. One of our survivor friends says that she has to be careful how much she listens to people because she can become nauseous when having to concentrate on someone else.
9. Plan in advance what you will wear and what you may need to take with you. Make a list or write notes on your phone or use sticky notes to remind yourself. This keeps you from feeling last-minute pressure that makes it difficult to function.
10. Keep things as simple as possible. This means simplifying decorations and meal planning as well as prioritizing what is important. Eliminating extra tasks and responsibilities helps reduce stress and unneeded sensory stimulation.

When planning to leave for an event, consider time frame reminders. A time frame reminder can be communicating something like a 30-minute window of arrival. It takes the pressure off the survivor and care partner. Or, sharing in a kind tone of, "Five minutes until you have to leave." It may be helpful to give a short directive such as, "Please start your shower." Perhaps the momentum of the shower will carry your survivor towards being ready to go to the event.

Moving is another one of those events that is very taxing. As a survivor, there are some considerations that may help the process. For example, assign as much packing as possible to another, be it a friend, a family member, or a moving company. Remember that unpacking normally falls on the person responsible for placing items. You may want to stay somewhere less chaotic until the move is completed. During the move, reduce outside obligations. Try not to overextend yourself with other outside responsibilities. Consider taking time off from work and other social events while you are in the process of moving. One of our TBI survivor friends took pictures of all of her things before the move. She said that she needed the pictures to remind her of what goes where. Along with pictures, consider writing down a list of to-dos and deadlines. An example of a to-do list: pack the dishes, call the moving company, call the electric company to initiate service. She also had an assistant (who understood the challenges of TBI) separate her household into three categories: things to donate, things to dispose of, things to move. The personal assistant can also help re-establish your house. Some survivors also code their tasks with color. For example, movers were given green. Utilities were given blue. And so on. Lastly, pace yourself according to your energy level (don't push yourself) as much as possible and plan for recovery time.

I know that the recovery of the brain is so often two steps forward, three steps back. And that brain injury is consistently inconsistent. However, I have confidence that you will experience steady improvement even when it doesn't feel like it. I wanted to give you a few travel tips to consider for your vacation. From what I have understood with other survivors, driving works better than flying unless it's a short flight. Consider stopping every one to two hours to walk, stretch, and grab a snack. Keep a casual schedule by not doing a lot of activities. Do something whimsical and fun. Macie, a TBI survivor, would talk with others at a restaurant or visitors' center. She said that it helped take her mind off the long trip. She said it gave her a breath of fresh air to visit with someone. Keep it simple. Perhaps schedule one big event each day instead of making yourself participate in three or four events. Please schedule rest during the vacation (think about taking a nap or going to your room for quiet time) and allow for rest days after you get back home. Again, let your care partner know if you are getting fatigued or need extra time to do things. Or, be OK with telling your caregiver that you need to rest and not participate in additional activities.

Participating in any family or community event is a BIG deal! For you to go and participate in an event is huge progress! Bottom line: plan, enjoy, and rest throughout the activity. Celebrate each event as a success because it is!

Happy for you!
Deana

Homework

- List two or three people who could be your travel buddy and/or your assistant.

  _____

  _____

- Develop an event plan that you could use next time you have an activity. For example, (1) rest before the event, (2) use earplugs and sunglasses, (3) schedule a rest day.

  _____

  _____

  _____

  _____

- Write down two activities that you will try during your next trip. For example, take pictures of scenery or neat moments or write posts on social media.

  _____

  _____

Resources

Rawlins, R. (2014). *Learning by accident: A caregiver's true story of fear, family, and hope.* Skyhorse Publishing.

Zellmer, A. (2018). *Embracing the journey: Moving forward after brain injury.* CreateSpace Independent Publishing Platform.

Meili, T. (2003). *I am the Central Park jogger: A story of hope and possibility.* Scribner.

12 Self-Esteem and Purpose

Self-Esteem

Brain injury can shake a person to the core. Because of the many life effects of the injury and the different levels of functioning, brain injury can fundamentally challenge a person in who they are and why they do what they do. It can redefine unique and personal qualities of who you are and your sense of self. Basically, brain injury reveals and shapes what you consider really important. It is a complex process to rediscover yourself and your purpose. Learning to live again after the injury "is an over-and-over process", according to Patti Foster (personal communication). It is trying to figure out "who he wants to be when he grows up". She further explains that there is no rhyme or reason in learning how to live again and be true to your heart after the basics of living have been snatched from a person.

Researchers talk about "self" as someone we know and with whom we are familiar. But what is the self or the person? Self can be a combination of personality, brain systems (how the brain works), cognition, and mental, social, emotional, and spiritual interactions. Some have said that the self is collective and consistent characteristics. There are several terms that sound similar but are different in definition. For example, self-efficacy is a person's evaluation about his ability to perform tasks. Self-concept is our thoughts and feelings about who we are and how we define ourselves. Self-awareness is the capacity to experience ourselves as distinct from others. And self-esteem is the judgement we make about our worth. I'm not trying to confuse you, but rather to show that there are distinctions for "self" throughout academia.

But what about brain injury survivors? All those previous definitions encompass the self, who you are. From my experience working with brain injury folks, self-esteem is where most struggle to redefine.

DOI: 10.4324/9781003602774-12

They have difficulty finding their worth or purpose post-injury. Research has shown that self-esteem improves with more participation in leisure activities and increased function. Basically, you feel better the more successfully you engage in fun and social activities. Whether the activity is a game of Uno or dinner with a friend. It boosts your confidence to participate. Although there is an initial decline, self-esteem can increase and stabilize with recovery. If there are depression and anxiety, self-esteem issues are more profound. So, when we work to redefine and understand our post-injury self, the possible mental health issues can improve.

Low Self-Esteem

What habits keep self-esteem low? Sometimes even when we do not want to, we can be too self-critical. We tend to put ourselves down when we make a mistake. A healthy dose of evaluating positives and negatives can be helpful. However, if we focus only on the negatives such as our faults and inabilities, the result is feeling worse about ourselves, our worth, and our ability to contribute to life. Being self-critical can contribute to helplessness and hopelessness. Do your best not to only focus on what you believe are flaws and weaknesses. Here are some signs that happen when someone has low self-esteem:

1. Withdrawal from social events. If you do not feel good about yourself, you usually will not want to be with others. For example, you would not go if you were invited for lunch.
2. Feeling unloved and unwanted. These feelings keep you from wanting to participate in relationships. Not feeling loved or wanted makes you feel bad about yourself and makes you unlikely to do anything with someone. It is a negative cycle.
3. Neglecting personal hygiene. Sometimes this is due to low energy, but it can also be due to low self-esteem. Make a list and start a routine of such things as brushing your teeth, combing your hair, putting on clean clothes, taking a bath.
4. Having negative self-talk. An example of this is, "Nobody wants to be my friend." Or, "I can't do anything right."
5. Inability to accept compliments. Whether you believe the compliment is true or not, say "thank you". It may be helpful for you to write down compliments you receive and put them in a journal. Maybe one day you will read the compliment and believe it!
6. Feeling shame, depressed, or anxious. There is a relationship between feeling shame, depressed, or anxious and having low self-

esteem. Consider talking to a trained professional counselor to help tackle these issues.

7   Trusting others too much. This comes with brain injury and believing people. The childlikeness and vulnerability of a newly brain-injured person set the stage for being overly trusting of others. This is a time when your caregiver can help you learn to trust someone appropriately. Also, as you learn to live again and learn more about yourself, you will develop a better sense of when someone can be trusted.

8   Poor motivation. The question that sometimes accompanies poor motivation is, "I don't know if I can." With brain injury, second-guessing and doubt can make you unsure of an outcome. That makes sense when you don't feel good about yourself or about any outcome. However, challenge that question and try to take a baby step towards progress. It will go a long way in helping you feel better about yourself.

What are some ways to recapture, recreate, or restore your self-esteem? Here are some suggestions that may be helpful:

1   Set simple goals for yourself. Accomplishing small goals sets the foundation for taking on bigger goals. For example, make a goal to write in your journal.

2   Be kind to yourself. This means allowing yourself space to make mistakes without criticizing yourself. It means not pushing yourself too hard or too fast. It means appreciating every effort. Say nice things to yourself. For example, saying "I am glad that I tried to wash my hair by myself."

3   Do not compare yourself to your pre-injury self. Oh my, this is a hard one! However, comparing yourself to others may give you a positive goal. It can encourage and motivate you to try something that they can do! For example, Patti volunteers at a local hospital unit of brain injury survivors. When they see her, they are encouraged that they too may be able to help others. They say, "If she can do it, maybe I can too. Let me try."

4   Increase time with others. In small ways, initiate conversations with someone. Simply asking a question or paying someone a compliment or saying thank you are good starts to a healthy social exchange. So many survivors want to give back after their injury. Visiting with others helps provide that opportunity.

5   Celebrate your wins. Every win deserves celebration! Learning to live again after sustaining a brain injury calls for you to appreciate every effort towards recovery.

It is my belief that we are all born in the image of God, the *Imago Dei*. Therefore, if we are created in God's image, then we have inherent worth. Some people think that their worth is connected to what they do. You are priceless simply because you are born. You are here. It is no accident. Life circumstances and tragedies cannot take that away. In fact, tragedy like brain injury can potentially be a catalyst for personal growth. So often I've seen survivors contribute to life in a more significant way than before the injury because they have a powerful story. A story that encourages others who are going through a tough time.

Our friend Rosa, Holocaust and TBI survivor, shared one of the ways that helped her survive challenges. She suffered a brain injury from being beaten with a baton by Josef Mengele in Auschwitz. She chose to see whatever happened to her as a benefit. For example, she said that the TBI helped her not fully understand the horrible things happening in the concentration camp. Rosa was intentional about seeing things in a positive light. This is one of several ways that people can improve their self-esteem. Even with the limitations of brain injury, there are some things that can be practiced that will improve how you feel about yourself and your relationships:

1 Listen. Listening to others helps them feel that you care. This sets a foundation for them to offer you the same gift of listening. For example, if your friend had a bad day. Ask her to tell you about it. Then listen to what she says and pay attention to how she says it. Do your best to not interrupt. Just listen.
2 Be gracious. Good manners call for us to be kind to others even when they make a mistake. This may mean forgiving someone who has wronged you. It could be offering to help someone in need. For example, you see someone struggling with their groceries, offering to help load them in their car. Graciousness is simply being kind, courteous, and generous in challenging situations.
3 Be attentive. Pay attention to the little things. This helps people know that you are interested in them. For example, celebrating someone who just signed their name when you know as a survivor that signing your name is hard!
4 Offer thanks. Gratitude is foundational to healthy relationships. For example, thanking your spouse for taking you to the doctor's office.
5 Spend time with positive people. Enjoying time with people who are optimistic offers a new perspective and healthy perspective on

life and its challenges. Happy people tend to make you feel good about yourself. For example, periodically Hope After Brain Injury hosts a movie/dinner night. We rent out a theatre and invite survivors and their families to have dinner and watch a movie. It is an evening of fun that helps everyone feel positive and happy that they can participate and have a good time.

Purpose

Faith practices or religions define purpose differently. The overall belief about purpose follows the moral and religious values of a certain faith. For example, Hinduism says purpose has three parts: righteous conduct and fulfilling one's duty in life while balancing desire and pleasure. Some eastern religions believe purpose is the escape from suffering and experiencing lasting peace. Other traditions emphasize understanding of one's own nature and its relationship with the universe. In western religions, purpose is glorifying God and living a life according to His will which includes having a relationship with Him as exhibited by belief and obedience. Atheism believes purpose is living in accordance with whatever the person believes it to be. Individuals are free to choose their own goals and meaning in life without relying on a divine purpose or creator. Whether you are faith-based or religious or not, you can choose what is fulfilling to you. Your purpose post-injury is a continuous process. You can decide what is important and meaningful and you can choose how you will share that with others.

Brain injury, depending on its severity, creates a disconnect between the life pre-injury and post-injury. Patti would say often, "I want to find my place in this world." So often survivors grieve for what they did prior to the injury and find it difficult to know what they can do after the injury. Sort of a battle between brokenness and ability. For some, purpose is found in participating in the workforce. Some survivors can return to their work that they were doing before the injury. Others find they enjoy volunteering. This gives them an opportunity to feel like they are making a difference. Whether you transition to a part-time or volunteer work schedule, it is a time to celebrate progress. This may be a time to work with a vocational rehabilitation (VR) counselor (if available). Their goal is to determine your skill level and abilities and help find work that best fits those abilities. As the survivor recovers and learns to manage the deficits, his ability to work improves.

As we addressed earlier in the book, the final stage of recovery is service. Most survivors try to come to terms with what has happened to them and do so through wanting to give back in some way. One survivor said that by living transparently, sharing his struggles and victories has given his life meaningful purpose. In the Christian faith, God's desire for us to be in relationship with Him does not change. In other words, no tragedy or circumstance can interrupt God's desire on someone's life. For many, brain injury helped reshape their purpose. His primary calling is for us to be in relationship to Him. For example, praying, reading the Bible, and attending services that help you understand God and His desires for you. The secondary calling or purpose is living out the relationship with the talents and gifts He has given, including the gifts and new insights that come from suffering. In other words, share with others what you have learned through brain injury. What words of wisdom can you provide that we need? Perhaps, it is human nature to want to share the suffering we have endured and how we have overcome the difficulty. Remember at the beginning of the book that I said you were this world's best-kept secret of resilience? This is what I mean. The world needs to hear your story and how you survived. What did you learn from it? Tell fellow survivors so the listener will have nuggets of wisdom and be able to navigate their tragedy. Please read Laura Stonitsch's poem written specifically for you. She shares her heart from her tragedy to you. (See appendix C.)

My belief is that no experience (negative or positive) is wasted if given to God. So, finding and living out purpose is life-giving to you and to those you love or those under your influence. To put it simply, you can make a difference in the lives of others! And interestingly, sometimes brain injury opens the door to new talents, gifts, and skills. Patti was formerly a radio personality. After her TBI, she became an author and international speaker. Cristabelle Braden began to write music after her brain injury as a teenager. She now hosts podcasts and facilitates support groups to help others going through brain injury recovery. Oliver Sacks wrote *Musicophilia* based on people who found a new talent after their brain injury. While I know that not everyone has a positive experience in their recovery, they can share their story which can encourage others to not give up. Our beloved TBI friend, Russ, did not have family support and was placed in an outside barn to live. Through an intervention, he was placed in a group home that gave him the love and support he needed. And although he could not always communicate clearly, you could very clearly hear him say, "I'm trying." He knew that he did not have a positive experience, yet he did his best to encourage us through not giving up.

The recovery process is a full-time job! Sometimes there are too many appointments in a week. It's OK to take a break and have a day to yourself. But do not stop prematurely. One way that helps people process their recovery is through writing. Consider beginning a journal that shares your struggles and strategies. Let's call it the "Struggles and Strategies Guide to Brain Injury Recovery". Let it be a place where you can write what you are dealing with and what you are doing to help. In other words, what coping strategy you are using. For example, you may forget to take your medicine (struggle). So you started to set alarms on your phone to remind you (strategy). Not only will this encourage you, but it will also be a guide to others. Plus, it will help your loved ones know how to help you more effectively. Every brain injury is different so your experience and strategies are priceless to your loved ones.

Letter to You

Dear Friend,

Finding yourself again after brain injury is a huge task! It is a self-discovery because you remember who you were but are in the process of learning who you are. Scott Farraway, a rehabilitation therapist in Canada, likes to refer to it as "recovery to discovery". I think that is a great way to understand the process of getting better. It is a perpetual discovery of who you are. Appreciate the differences between your previous self and current self but please don't compare. It's an inaccurate comparison and it typically leads to sadness, depression, and despair. I have found in private practice that survivors go through the grieving stage of missing who they were. That is completely understandable. But please don't stay there...in the missing (focusing on what you don't have). Do your best to also appreciate who you are now. Consider the strength, fortitude, and courage you have shown to survive a brain injury and to create a new life. You are amazing! A British friend of mine used to say, "They have a strong constitution." As a professional counselor, I have been impressed over and over again at survivors' ability to go forward. They have the courage to try what is scary (learning to live again). They have the fortitude or stick-with-it-ness to not give up. They have the strength to keep going. That's a strong constitution! Whether people tell you or not, they are looking at you and what you have gone through. They are in awe of you as well. (Those that are not do not belong in your sphere of support. You need to be surrounded by cheerleaders, not criticizers.) Recognize the growth as it balances the loss. Just like your "checkbook"...TBI made some serious withdrawals, but you are working hard to make deposits! When thinking about losing ground or momentum, please also consider the gains. It's just not fair to only evaluate one side. You deserve a fair evaluation! The progress of brain injury recovery is staggered like there is no rhyme or reason to it. For example, your balance may improve, but your memory may not. You may be more fluent, but your mood fluctuates. It's kind of mean that way. But if you can look through a long lens instead of a zoom lens, you will notice progress in the process. You've done extremely well these several years! I'm proud of you.

Creating an edited self takes time and reflection. One thing I suggest in trying to find yourself again is start with the basic questions. Like, what's your favorite color? What food do you like now? The basics help direct you to the deeper things. You may find that your likes and dislikes have changed since the injury. For example, Sally said that she used to like spicy food but since her TBI she prefers blander meals. Drue said that since the wreck, she does not have any taste at all so she eats "from memory". Meaning, she eats what she knows she liked before her TBI. Maybe before brain injury someone enjoyed detective shows but now they enjoy animation. Use the time to discover the new refined you. And do your best to not judge it as good or bad. It simply is a new experience of yourself. Also, think about your interests and what you enjoy or want to enjoy. As you get better, you will have more energy and more clarity. You will understand things about yourself that never changed from the injury. You may not need as many naps. You will also learn where to direct your physical and cognitive energy. Your refined self will shine more brightly! I would like to suggest you come up with a list that describes who you are now. Here are some examples:

1 Your processor is sometimes slower, but you come to the right conclusion. (Some have described their brain as a computer that has a slower processor.)
2 You are competent.
3 You are kind, respectful, courageous.
4 You are a wonderful mom, dad, sibling, spouse, child, parent, co-parent, caregiver.
5 You are a great friend.
6 Your heart is not injured. It is full of love and tenderness.
7 You usually enjoy small gatherings instead of big parties.
8 You are doing the best that you can.

Hang on to those truths and come up with a few of your own. What would you add to this list? Here's a reminder...your spirit does not have TBI. Another example: "You are a beautiful soul that no injury can diminish."

New identity...I am thankful that you are embracing this opportunity to recreate yourself and your life after brain injury. It is a culmination of grief, celebration, and anticipation. In other words, recovery means recognizing what is lost, celebrating what you have, and being excited about your future. Part of recovery is shedding the shame of abuse. A tough topic here. But there are times when survivors experience physical, verbal, and emotional abuse from others. This is not the survivor's fault. In fact, they are more vulnerable because they do not have the capacity to protect themselves. After Lisa's accident, she struggled with feeling dizzy. Her husband would intentionally do things that made that worse. Our friend Russ (mentioned above) was neglected and physically beaten. The result of abuse can make the survivor feel shame, like they caused it or could have prevented it, or simply not understand why it happened. The truth is that they were and are innocent. As a professional counselor, we work together to help the survivor understand what happened and how to process those feelings of shame. If you know of anyone in an abusive or neglectful environment, please contact emergency services in your area.

The challenge in recovery is using the time to heal and create. The treatment involved in recovery can be demanding of your time and space to heal. But try to carve out a few minutes to sit outside (weather permitting) and soak up the sun. Allow your body and brain to relax. You may find that refreshment helps you feel rested, and even creative. There are so much freedom and creativity in using one's voice. The Lord created the universe with His voice. And you have power in your voice! Your voice is saying things like "yes" or "no" or "I prefer". It is giving yourself permission to try. Saying nice things to yourself and encouraging others are two more examples of using your voice. I want you to speak life into yourself. This is important because many survivors lost their voice (their ability to speak) in the accident. Regaining the ability to use your voice, to communicate, even if it is nonverbal, is a huge step in creating the life you want. The strength of your voice is in defense and offense. God is giving you a new life experience. Using your voice gives you the opportunity to create a life that best suits you now.

When thinking about loss, it's a soft hand-off between grief and purpose. What I mean is that when we grieve what we have lost, we automatically turn to what we have. We tend to think about how the past can help us in the future. Ask yourself what you learned from the tragedy and how you want to take those lessons into the future. You have survived and now you are in the process of living and thriving. Trouble is, life will look different and eerily the same. Let's say that you know you love plants. Now, you get to introduce them back into your life in a manner that works with your energy level. Contributing to someone's life is important to you. The great news is that there are no rules...well, except to not hurt yourself. You get to co-create with God. Ask Him what He wants and watch for Him to make the way.

Finding your purpose...that's hard because you are in the process of learning to live again. Moving towards relationships and moving away from things that create pressure are super-helpful in recovery. I believe God has given you a bigger mission field. Living each day as well as you are able can be your purpose. An example of contributing to the community is working with the children at church, which can be considered HUGE purpose! And btw, most TBI folks enjoy kids much better than adults! Your "why" is deeper now. Your gut is directing you towards health. Listen to it. I'm glad you are considering using the voice God gave you. It's imperative for continued health. We tend to silence ourselves to find peace but, in the end, we sacrifice ourselves. That may be necessary for a short time, but not life-giving for a long time. An example is, if your spouse is driving too fast, you stay silent to keep from having an argument. But after a few speedy rides, the nervousness and uneasiness become too much. By not saying something (like "please slow down"), you sacrifice yourself. Hope that makes sense. My recommendation is for you to say something if you are uncomfortable. Others may not know if you don't tell them. You've been at death's door. You know what it's like to lose almost everything. You are like a phoenix who comes out of the fire to soar again. You have come through the gauntlet of tragedy and are learning to live again! Your presence offers hope to others. Let's not put ourselves in a box of expectations, what we should do or what others expect. Let's open ourselves to the ministry God has called us to. It's His responsibility to reveal it to you. Your brain has been injured, but not your Spirit. In fact, you have a closer relationship with God because of the suffering you've been through. One last thing...there may be times when you feel disconnected to God. Like He is as far away as the next universe. Be OK with that. It's simply a statement of energy and resources, not a reflection of your spiritual relationship. One of the strongest prayers I read was from Corrie ten Boom, a Holocaust survivor. She was in solitary confinement and physically ill. Her prayer was, "God, if I can stand up today. Let that be my prayer to you." I am reminded of a great promise in Psalm 28:7 (New International Version) which says, "The Lord is my strength and my shield." Remember that the Almighty is on your side helping you along the way. Also, use wisdom as a coping strategy for recovery and loss. Being wise is managing what you can without pushing yourself to do more. Wisdom allows you to rest and move forward with grace. Wisdom is kind and gentle, especially to someone grieving, in recovery. Thank you for moving away from positions that create pressure and moving towards relationships.

In brain injury recovery, feeling insecure comes with the territory. I have heard TBI survivors say, "I never doubted myself or second-guessed myself until the brain injury." There is nothing wrong with your IQ. The processing speed has slowed. I think one of the hardest things about brain recovery is that it's hard to trust your brain. Questions like, "Am I seeing that right? Did I understand that correctly?" are forever in your head. When those questions come, rest in your gut. It will tell you the truth, the direction. It's not brain-injured. Your spirit is not brain-injured. Remember that brain injury affects your brain and your body, but it does not affect your heart or spirit. Those are still intact and very alive. It can be difficult to be confident with one thing and doubtful about something else. Believe it or not, that's part of healing. The brain doesn't heal at the same rate in the same place. Please know that when you feel more anchored, you will excel again. Feeling anchored is about feeling more secure in yourself and in your brain. Practicing coping strategies that you learned in your therapies will help you feel more anchored. Trying to do something that you haven't been able to before will help you feel more confident. In the meantime, rest, listen to uplifting podcasts, read poetry, or do whatever brings you peace and joy.

Thinking of strategies to help you function, consider these statements. Perhaps you can add to the list and write some of your own strategies!

1 Be extra gentle with myself especially after a long, emotional, or cognitively challenging day. For example, allow yourself to rest and do not push yourself to do more.
2 Regression is to be expected. Don't build your house on it. Meaning, know that regression is a stage, not a destination. It tends to be the nature of brain injury too. You may have success in remembering something one day and the next not remember it at all. Just know that's part of the recovery. It is not because you are not trying. You are doing the best that you can.

3   "Slow and steady" is a new mantra (short phrase you can repeat to yourself). Remember the children's story, "The Tortoise and the Hare"? The slow and steady tortoise was more successful than the fast-moving hare that was too tired to finish first.
4   Wisdom says to not push. Please be wise with your energy (physical, cognitive, and emotional). I've noticed that when survivors are most fatigued, they tend to push themselves and tend to make more mistakes. It is OK to rest and to move at a slower pace.
5   Be nice to my brain by creating reminder lists. This might mean having a whiteboard in your kitchen that has all your appointments on them. It may mean creating a notebook with daily chores. A speech therapist friend suggests to use pens that have erasers on them so if you make a mistake or the plans change, you can erase the entry and make it right.

In the end, TBI will be a part of your story, but it will never be your whole story. You are greater than your injury. And more importantly, God is greater than brain injury. Your worth is not measured by productivity. Your worth is because you were made in the image of God (the *Imago Dei*). You are healing. Crawling is still moving. You are on your way to walking and running!

Be encouraged, dear Friend. Brain injury has expanded your influence. Your injury has allowed you to help people in a way you may not have envisioned. It has deepened your faith. It has given you the opportunity to recreate yourself and embrace your purpose. However long you feel like your life stopped for, remember that you are in the process of creating an impactful future. Choose life. Choose health. Choose purpose. You'll be glad you did.

Excited for your future,
Deana

Homework

- Write down four compliments you have received. For each compliment, how did it make you feel? What did it make you think?

_____

_____

_____

_____

- List two struggles and two strategies that help you manage the struggle.

  _____

  _____

- Tell about at least two people or two things that helped you discover your purpose.

  _____

  _____

- What are two things that you most appreciate about your purpose?

  _____

  _____

Resources

Braden, C. (2017). *More to me: Discovering your freedom through identity.* CreateSpace Independent Publishing Platform.

Sacks, O. (2008). *Musicophilia: Tales of music and the brain* (revised and expanded edition). Vintage.

Foster, P. (2020). *Coping with traumatic brain injury: One woman's journey from death to life.* Redemption Press.

Appendix A
Visualization – Cloud

Begin by finding a relaxed and comfortable position, either lying down or sitting, in a place where you will not be interrupted.
Take a deep breath through your abdomen, hold it for a few seconds, and exhale slowly. As you breathe, notice your stomach rising and your lungs filling with air.
Breathe in 1…2…3, hold…2…3. And exhale…2…3. Slowly feel your body become more and more relaxed. As you exhale, imagine the tension leaving your body and drifting out of the room…
Inhale…2…3 and exhale…2…3
Feel your body releasing all the tension, all the stress, becoming relaxed, calm, and peaceful.
Feel the weight of your body and the limpness of your arms and legs.
A quiet wave of relaxation is flowing from your head, down to your neck, shoulders, chest, back, arms, hands, legs, and feet.
Inhale…2…3 and exhale…2…3
Imagine yourself breathing in fresh energy and oxygen that is flowing through your whole body.
Notice a white cloud entering your awareness. Now imagine yourself floating on that soft billowy white cloud. The cloud is slowly lifting you from where you are resting and is holding you in the air. You begin to feel lighter as you sink into the softness of the white fluffy cloud. As you lie in the cloud, you begin to notice how comfortable you are becoming. As your body relaxes, your tension melts away.
Inhale…2…3 and exhale…2…3
You feel yourself floating into the clear blue sky, feeling the warmth of the sun and the coolness of the breeze…a perfect temperature.
Notice your body touching the cloud, how soft it feels, the softness of how it feels floating on air, swaying gently with the wind. You feel safe, relaxed, calm.

You begin to let yourself rest in the soft support of the cloud. As you look around, you notice other clouds in the sky, illuminated by the sun as they float gently by. You take a moment to enjoy their presence.
As you float higher and higher, you breathe in the clean fresh air.
Inhale...2...3 and exhale...2...3
You feel totally relaxed, noticing how peaceful the sky is, how calm it is, how quiet.
Imagine the green grass below, gently blowing in the wind. The grass recedes farther as you rise into the sky. The grass looks like a soft green carpet, the wind creating gentle waves as if it were water.
Imagine the trees reaching to meet you with their leaves whispering in the soft breeze. Imagine the scent of soft rain in the distance and the scent of sweet flowers from the neighboring hills.
Inhale....2...3 and exhale....2...3
Continue floating through the air on your soft, comfortable, peaceful cloud. Drifting...as high as you wish.
The ground below looks like a giant patchwork of green grass and flowers of all colors...yellow, pink, blue, green, purple, and red. Patches of lakes and rivers slowly moving through the hills.
Feel the cloud beneath you...supporting you smoothly and comfortably.
Feel the freedom to float wherever you wish. You can look down on forests, the countryside, snow-covered mountains or drift alongside an ocean...float wherever you like.
Inhale...2...3 and exhale...2...3
Enjoy the sights around you. Enjoy floating on a cloud. You are relaxed and peaceful...
Now, when you are ready and only when you are ready, allow your cloud to drift back towards the earth. Let your cloud bring you back into your day calmly and peacefully.
Imagine your cloud becoming part of where you are resting. Feel the surface where you are sitting or lying down. Imagine the cloud slowly disappearing as the real surface becomes more solid beneath you.
Inhale...2...3 and exhale...2...3
You begin to slowly and gently bring your attention back to the room, still feeling relaxed and comfortable. Continue to rest for another few moments.
Slowly, open your eyes. Feel your body relaxed and refreshed. See your surroundings. Move your arms and legs. Turn your head. And when you are ready – only when you are ready – return to your day feeling relaxed, refreshed, and calm from your journey on a cloud.

Appendix B
Outside, Inside

      On the outside
You see me as normal
On the inside
I see how non-normal I am.
      On the outside
I appear involved in the discussion
On the inside
I see how furiously my brain is working – just to keep up.
      On the outside
You see me forget things
On the inside
I am infuriated by my forgetfulness.
      On the outside
My words seem to come easily
On the inside
I can feel the words slipping away from my lips.
      On the outside
You see me laughing at jokes
On the inside
I don't get it – I feel stupid.
      On the outside
You see me as normal
On the inside
I see my brain injury
And it hurts.

                        Courtesy by Jan Gazda, TBI survivor

Appendix C
Brain Injury Survivor Poem

Brain Injury Survivor,

Every brain injury is unique; no injury is the same. You may struggle with balance, vision, and/or remembering names. You may fatigue quickly and struggle with pain. You may feel alone, maybe even ashamed.

But survivor, I'm here to congratulate you. I know that brain injuries aren't easy to get through. I want you to know that I celebrate you. You are a fighter; I know this is true!

God, I pray that you give each survivor hope. Holy Spirit, comfort them, and help them cope. I pray for healing, encouragement, peace, and love to invade, each person who reads this letter today.

I can't say I understand everything you are going through. But I'm writing to you as someone who has had brain surgeries and several complications, too. My life's been disrupted so many times. I've asked God many questions, including why?

I've spent years in recovery, been in wheelchairs, and couldn't do anything except lie in bed. Nothing seemed to help ease the pain in my head. But the pain wasn't just physical; it hurt mentally, emotionally, and spiritually, too. People didn't seem to understand the hidden pain was often the most difficult to get through.

I want to encourage you to keep fighting and not quit. Sometimes it may feel like it's hit after hit. But survivor, I encourage you to find hope in Jesus Christ. He knows your pain; His truth dismantles lies.

For years, I thought I must have done something wrong. Why else would this hardship last for so long? I don't have the answers as to why some suffer more than others. But I love you survivor, sister and brother.

I encourage you to find something to be grateful for today. My favorite thing is Satan can't take my relationship with God away! You have a purpose to live; God's not mad at you. Survivor, keep going; I'm proud of you!

Courtesy by Laura Stonitsch, LPCA (TX), CCC-SLP

References

Adams, D. (2023). *Christian and faith-based counseling for brain injury: Techniques for survivors and families.* Routledge.
Cassidy, J. (2009). *Mindstorms: The complete guide for families living with traumatic brain injury.* De Capo Press.
Coetzer, R. (2018). *Anxiety and mood disorders following traumatic brain injury: Clinical assessment and psychotherapy.* Routledge.
Curvis, W., & Methley, A. (Eds.). (2022). *Acceptance and commitment therapy and brain injury: A practical guide for clinicians.* Routledge.
Darmofal, K. (2015). *101 tips for recovering from traumatic brain injury: Practical advice for TBI survivors, caregivers, and teachers.* Loving Healing Press.
Denton, G. (2008). *Brainlash: Maximize your recovery from mild traumatic brain injury* (3rd ed.). Demos.
Elliott, C. (2016). *The ghost in my brain: How a concussion stole my life and how the new science of brain plasticity helped me get it back.* Penguin Books.
Feasel, C., & Yorkey, M. (2016). *After the cheering stops: An NFL wife's story of concussions, loss, and the faith that saw her through.* Thomas Nelson.
Fins, J. (2015). *Rights come to mind: Brain injury, ethics, and the struggle of consciousness.* Cambridge University Press.
Gordon, C. (2018). *Turn the lights on!: A physician's personal journey from the darkness of traumatic brain injury (TBI) to hope, healing, and recovery.* Corpus Callosum Creations.
Huxford, J. (2018). *Finding normal: An uninvited change, an unexpected outcome.* Morgan James Faith.
Klonoff, P. (2010). *Psychotherapy after brain injury: Principles and techniques.* The Guilford Press.
Klonoff, P. (2024). *Holistic neurorehabilitation: Interventions to support functional skills after acquired brain injury.* The Guilford Press.
Lassaletta, A. (2020). *The invisible brain injury: Cognitive impairments in traumatic brain injury, stroke, and other acquired brain pathologies.* Routledge.

References

Lawton, S. (2016). *Head first! A crash course in positivity.* Fedd Books.

Lewis, S. (2010). *Rise and shine: The extraordinary story of one man's journey from near death to full recovery.* Santa Monica Press.

Liontas, A. (2024). *Sex with a brain injury: On concussion and recovery.* Scribner.

Mandrell, B., & Vecsey, G. (1990). *Get to the heart: My story.* Bantam.

Mason, M. (2009). *Head cases: Stories of brain injury and its aftermath.* Farrar, Straus, and Giroux.

McCrea, M. (2008). *Mild traumatic brain injury and postconcussion syndrome: New evidence base for diagnosis and treatment.* Oxford University Press.

Ownsworth, T. (2014). *Self-identity after brain injury.* Psychology Press.

Ponsford, J., Sloan, S., & Snow, P. (2012). *Traumatic brain injury: Rehabilitation for everyday adaptive living* (2nd ed.). Psychology Press.

Ruff, R., & Chester, S. (2014). *Effective psychotherapy for individuals with brain injury.* The Guilford Press.

Slott, P., & Spears, M. (2015). *Damage control: A brain injury survivor helps you beat the odds.* CreateSpace Independent Publishing Platform.

Stoler, D., & Hill, B. (1998). *Coping with mild traumatic brain injury: A guide to living with the challenges associated with concussion/brain injury.* Avery.

Swanson, K. (1999). *I'll carry the fork! Recovering a life after brain injury.* Rising Star Press.

Tuttle, K. (2023). *After the crash: How to keep your job, stay in school, live life after a brain injury.* Running Paws Publishing.

Valentino, D. (2013). *Headstrong: Surviving a traumatic brain injury without losing my mind.* Brown Books Publishing.

Valentino, D. (2016). *Heartstrong: Overcome obstacles and live life to the fullest.* Inspire on Purpose Publishing.

Vasterling, J. (2012). *PTSD and mild traumatic brain injury* (R. Bryant & T. Keane, Eds.). The Guilford Press.

Winslade, W. (1998). *Confronting traumatic brain injury: Devastation, hope, and healing.* Yale University Press.

Ziglar, Z., & Norman, J. (2013). *Embracing the struggle: Living life on life's terms.* Howard Books.

Zollman, F. (Ed.). (2021). *Manual of traumatic brain injury: Assessment and management* (3rd ed.). Demos Medical.

Index

ABI *see* Acquired Brain Injury (ABI)
academic skills deficits 15–16
Acquired Brain Injury (ABI) 6
agitation 16, 69, 79–80
all-or-nothing thinking 101
ambiguous grief 33, 60, 96
ambiguous loss 33, 88, 92, 96, 109; *see also* grief
amygdala 4–5, 12, 126
anger 32, 64, 89; and brain injury 64–5; coping strategies 68–72; levels of 65; management 67–8; triggers 65–7
anosognosia *see* lack of awareness
anxiety 45–6; caregivers 36; cognitive restructuring 51; loss 46–7; management 47–51, 52–3; mindfulness 48; progressive muscle relaxation 50; recovery after TBI 46–7; relaxation techniques 50; tactical breathing technique 48; three great losses 46; travel 126–7; "Visualization–Cloud" 50
auditory overload 113–14
autonomic nervous system 4

Beethoven, L. van 55
Boss, P. 88, 92
Braden, C. 140
brain 1; amygdala 4–5; cerebellum 1, 2, 19; cerebral cortex 1; cerebrum 1; corpus callosum 2; frontal lobe 3–4; hippocampus 5; hypothalamus 4; medulla oblongata 6; myelin 2; occipital lobe 2; parietal lobe 3; pineal gland 6; pituitary gland 5; pons 6; prefrontal cortex 3; stem 1; temporal lobe 3; thalamus 4
brain injury 6–8; embracing life after 141–6; message to survivors 152; non-traumatic brain injury 6–7; survivor poem 151; traumatic brain injury 7–10; vision issues after 126–7

catastrophizing 57, 101
CBT *see* cognitive-behavioral therapy (CBT)
cerebellum 1, 2, 19
cerebral cortex 1
cerebrum 1
Churchill, W. 55
cognitive-behavioral therapy (CBT) 71, 57, 101
cognitive distortions 57–8, 101–2
cognitive processing therapy (CPT) 102
cognitive restructuring 51
concussion 7
confabulation 33, 85
containment 95
coordination and balance 19
corpus callosum 2
CPT *see* cognitive processing therapy (CPT)

DAI *see* diffuse axonal injury (DAI)
David, King 59, 93

deficits 12, 122; academic challenges 15–16; coordination and balance 19; coping strategies 22–9, 33; filter absence 24; flooding 14–15; impulsivity 17–19; irritability and agitation 79–80; lack of awareness 17–19; mood swings 16–17; personality changes 19–21; rigid thinking 21–2; short-term memory loss 12–14, 86
depression 55, 65, 89, 93; and brain injury 58–9; caregivers 36; cognitive-behavioral therapy 57; cognitive distortions 57–8; managing depression 57–8; support and coping strategies 59–62; symptoms 56–7; "talk therapy" 58
Descartes 6
dhyana 123
diffuse axonal injury (DAI) 8
discounting the positive 101
disinhibition *see* impulsivity
distress 103

Elliott, H. 89
EMDR *see* eye movement desensitization and processing (EMDR)
emotional overload 115
energy conservation 107, 115–16, 131
eustress *see* good stress
events 125; coping strategies and support 130; holidays 125–6; sporting events 129–30; survival guide 130–3; travel 126–8; worship gatherings 129
external sensory input 24
eye movement desensitization and processing (EMDR) 101

family 9, 31; adaptation 33–4; anger 64; impact of brain injury 34–7; care partner's strength 37–43; disillusionment 31–2; grief and ambiguous loss 91–3; lack of assistance 56; mourning 32–3; recovery stages 31–4; service 34; stress 103; survival 31; therapy 71; *see also* relationships
Farraway, S. 141

fatigue 23, 66, 79, 112, 129, 130; auditory overload 113–14; decision-fatigue 120; emotional overload 115; energy conservation 115–16; heart 120; management 117–20; physical overload 114–15; psychology of recovery 120–3; signals of 116–17; therapy 10; visual overload 114
fikr 123
flooding 14–15, 24, 122, 129
Foster, P. 26, 33, 42, 50, 69, 77, 85, 86, 90, 100, 116, 117, 125, 128, 135, 137, 139, 140
frontal lobe 3–4, 17, 24, 64, 77

Gage, P. 20
gezellig 131
Gogh, V. van 55
"good grief" 95
good stress 103
grief 32, 88, 109; ambiguous 60, 88, 90–1, 96; caregiver's perspective 91–3; emotional complexity and lack of closure 91–3; "good grief" 95; healing after loss and trauma 93–6; Kübler-Ross' five stages of 88, 89, 93; -related sadness 57; survivor's perspective 90–1
guided cloud meditation 149–50

Harrison Warren, T. 95
The Hiding Place (ten Boom) 131
hippocampus 5, 12
holidays 107, 125–6, 130–3
homeostasis 4
hypersensitivity 24
hypothalamus 4

implicit memory 12, 52
impulsivity 17–19
inflexible or rigid thinking 21–2
invisible injury *see* traumatic brain injury

Jesus Christ 8, 59

Kennedy, J. F. 122
koan 122
Kübler-Ross, E. 88, 89

lack of awareness 17–19
limbic system 4, 64–5
Lincoln, A. 55
"little brain" *see* cerebellum
long-term memory 22
loss 46–7
loss of consciousness 7
Love Your Brain 19

Maas, A. 50
meditation 50–1, 122–3, 149–50
medulla oblongata 6
melancholia *see* depression
memory 12; explicit 12; hippocampus 5; implicit 12, 52; long-term 22; loss 7, 12–14, 23, 100; motor 12; short-term 12–14, 22, 75; working 12
Mengele, J. 51, 138
mindfulness 9, 48, 69, 109
mood swings 16–17, 59
Musicophilia (Sacks) 140
myelin 2

Necessary Losses (Viorst) 94
neuroplasticity 9, 22, 23, 32, 60
neurotransmitters 106
Newton, I. 55
non-traumatic brain injury (NTBI) 6–7
NTBI *see* non-traumatic brain injury (NTBI)

occipital lobe 2
orbitofrontal lobe 65
overgeneralization 57, 101

pacing 26, 117–18, 121, 128, 130
parietal lobe 3, 15, 17, 20
Parton, D. 55
perseveration *see* inflexible or rigid thinking
personality changes 19–21
personalization 101, 102
Phelps, M. 55
physical overload 114–15
pineal gland 6
pituitary gland 5
pons 6
post-traumatic amnesia 7

post-traumatic stress 100
Prayer in the Night (Warren) 95
prefrontal cortex 3, 12
progressive muscle relaxation 50, 69
psychoeducation 71
purpose 83, 90–1, 139–41, 144

recovery 10, 23
"recovery to discovery" 141–6
relationships 74, 107; impact of brain injury 34–7; colleagues and acquaintances 82–3; communication 75, 77, 79; friendships 81–2; parenting 78–80; partners 74–8; rebuilding 38; siblings 80–1; strategies and support for caregivers 83–6; *see also* family
relaxation techniques 50, 69, 104, 115
retrograde amnesia 7
rigid thinking *see* inflexible or rigid thinking
Rowling, J. K. 55

Sacks, O. 140
St. Thomas 8
self 135; -awareness 21, 135; -compassionate strategies 145–6; -concept 135; -efficacy 135; -regulation 18
self-esteem 45, 135; low self-esteem 136–7; rebuilding 137–9
sensory overload 14, 113, 126–30
serotonin 61, 106
short-term memory loss (STM loss) 12–14, 86
STM loss *see* short-term memory loss (STM loss)
Stonitsch, L. 140, 152
stress 99, 102; coping strategies for stressful events 125–6; distress 103; emotional overload 115; good stress or eustress 103; handling 103–5, 115; psychological barriers and pathways to healing 105–9; remedy for 25; and sensory challenges 126–8; symptoms of 103; *see also* anxiety
support groups 9, 35–6, 49, 71, 81

tactical breathing technique 48
"talk therapy" 36, 58

TBI *see* traumatic brain injury (TBI)
temporal lobe 3
ten Boom, C. 131, 144
thalamus 4
"therapy fatigue" 10
trauma 99, 100; post-traumatic stress 100; psychological barriers and pathways to healing 105–9; source of 100; therapy 101–2
traumatic brain injury (TBI) 6, 7, 64, 99, 100; causes of 8; memory loss after 13; shifting roles and relationships after 34–7; survivor's encouragement 8–10; types of 7–8

travel 28, 126–8, 130–3

vestibular therapy 19
Viorst, J. 94
"Visualization–Cloud" 50, 149–50
visual overload 114
vocational rehabilitation counsellor (VR counsellor) 83, 139
VR counsellor *see* vocational rehabilitation counsellor (VR counsellor)

worship gatherings 129

yearning 91

For Product Safety Concerns and Information please contact our EU representative GPSR@taylorandfrancis.com
Taylor & Francis Verlag GmbH, Kaufingerstraße 24, 80331 München, Germany

www.ingramcontent.com/pod-product-compliance
Lightning Source LLC
Chambersburg PA
CBHW051542230426
43669CB00015B/2693